Views from the Podium

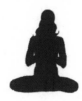

The life & times of a hot yogi

Tori Hicks-Glogowski

For the heroes in my life:

My Mom & Dad,

Jeffrey,

&

Jane

CONTENTS

INTRODUCTION

The mission of this book is to inspire yoga students to continue to come back to their mats, day after day, as is the mission of my blog by the same name. This book was meant to serve two different kind of readers. First, it is a memoir. It is my journey with the yoga and the book can be read cover to cover as most people read any story. Second, it was meant for the student waiting for class to begin at their yoga studio. In between each chapter, the reader will find short vignettes from a small sampling of my students that have had great success within their practice that ultimately affected their life in a profoundly positive way. Also, included are a collection of the most well-received blog posts that have been published to the blog over the last five years. These quick reads are intended to give the reader a small shot of inspiration before they make their way into the hot room for their daily yoga class.

This book is a snapshot of my life. My thoughts on life, and yoga, continue to evolve each day, as do the perceptions of my past. To state the obvious, this is one person's opinion of the people around them and as close to my truth as I can get. Some names and subtle facts have been changed as the focus of the story is on my own experiences and I wish to protect the privacy of those involved. Their stories aren't mine to tell.

PROLOGUE

This Is How Yoga Works...

From the Blog: April 30, 2013

You see a sign outside a storefront or an advertisement on the web or in a local paper and you think, "I should really give that yoga stuff a try." Your best friend's sister's cousin swears by it. Your doctor or chiropractor has told you it might be a good idea. And wasn't one of your friends going on and on about it a couple of weeks ago? But for some reason, in this moment, you are drawn to it more than at any other time.

The first class is a challenge. The postures, the teacher, the heat — all of it feels ridiculously impossible. You sit out half the class wondering why you came. Each posture you make it through brings a realization of the flexibility you lack or the strength you would need to go further. You walk out thinking, "That was rough. Maybe yoga isn't for me."

But later that day you feel amazing. You have never felt so relaxed or open. Your mind has never felt so quiet. This is the yoga working. This is when you know you have to go back.

You start a regular practice and actually look forward to the days you know you can take class. This is not because you feel incredible during the class — in fact, you are sweaty, hot, and sometimes in pain. Afterwards, though, you feel unstoppable.

A couple of months pass. Friends and family start to notice how great you look. It's not just that you have lost some weight and gained some muscle tone. Your skin also looks clearer and more vibrant. You are happier. Everyday anxieties and worries seem to roll off of your back. You have a confidence that is noticeable and enviable.

People begin asking you what you are doing differently. You tell them about the yoga classes you are taking. In fact, you can't *stop* talking about the yoga. Somehow, in just a few short months it has become part of who you are.

You have more energy. This is when you begin volunteering for a favorite organization, you start spending more time with your family, you become more effective at work, or you have true quality time with your friends. Smiling at others and performing random acts of kindness are part of your daily routine. You are able to think about others because you are no longer concerned solely with yourself. You are already taking care of yourself at the yoga studio.

Your friends and family start thinking about taking a yoga class based on your results. They go through their first classes and start a regular practice. You are directly affecting your community just by taking a yoga class a couple of times a week.

Your practice grows stronger and is an inspiration to those who practice with you and those who teach you. You become a teacher through example.

You may even discover that you are among the yoga practitioners who get an itch to share the yoga on a broader scale. They daydream about becoming yoga teachers. Eventually, they make the choice to go to teacher training. As they train, they are challenged on new levels, but they can't imagine not leading a class and find the sacrifices required to become a teacher completely worth it.

They come home and teach. Watching others discover the yoga and benefits it has on their lives has become thrilling and engaging. They lend their own strengths and talents to each class to assist their students through the process. As they teach, they continue on their own path of self-discovery. The more they learn, the more they can share with others.

Some of these teachers even dream of opening their own studios. Not to be in charge, but to directly affect an entire community that may not know about the yoga yet. They find a location to open a studio, put signs outside their storefronts, and advertise on the web or in the local paper to help others find the yoga.

That's when someone sees the sign or the ad and thinks, "I should really give that yoga stuff a try...."

CHAPTER ONE

A SWEATY START

The glowing sign on the side of an old brick building, "BikramYoga" in blue letters lined with red and orange flames, captured my attention immediately. A hot yoga studio. I had seen a story about this yoga on the local news a few weeks before. The practitioners that were interviewed had been soaked in sweat, red faced, and to my surprise, grinning from ear to ear as they discussed the benefits of this workout fad that seemed to be growing in popularity.

When I had been performing in a show in Pennsylvania about six months before, two of my cast members had gone to one of these classes. They had returned to the cast house, red cheeked and smiling as they described the intensity of the class to the bleary-eyed actors lounging on the sofa and sipping on their first cups of coffee for the day. At the time, I didn't pay much attention, since the show would be closing in less than a week. My focus then was on going home to my husband, Jeffrey, and working to get the next show booked, not on taking a yoga class. But the thought of trying a hot yoga class had stayed with me. It sounded different from what I thought a regular yoga class would be, everyone stretching for hours on end with no real "workout" happening. At least I would sweat in hot yoga.

I pointed the sign out to Jeffrey as we crossed the street and turned the corner. It was a balmy August evening in 2005, and we were exploring the downtown area of our new home, the suburbs of Chicago. We had just moved back the week before after five long years in the Quad Cities, on the border of Illinois and Iowa. Jeffrey would be starting his new job as a middle school music teacher.

"You want to take a yoga class?" he asked.

"It's a *hot* yoga class. The room is heated so that you sweat more than usual. I think it might be fun."

"When are you going to find the time to go? Most days you're booked from the moment you wake up until you go to bed."

He was referring to my dance classes and voice lessons and auditions and the temp jobs I took between theater gigs. It was a constant juggling act to keep everything balanced, and it was a rare moment when I would find myself with "free time." Still, I thought, it would be a nice break to do something that had nothing to do with my career.

"Oh, I don't know, but I'll try it someday," I vowed. "It's good to know we have a studio close by and now I know where it is."

About a month later I found my opportunity. One day after work at my current temp job, with no dance class, scene study class, or voice lesson to attend, I hurried home and dressed for my first attempt at hot yoga. As I put on a tank top and my favorite, black, flowy cotton capris, I thought of the dance audition I had on Thursday - maybe with all this so-called sweating and stretching I'd feel lighter and better equipped to deal with once again being in a leotard and high heels in front of strangers as I kicked and twirled my way into the next show.

Arriving at the studio, I opened the outside door and climbed the steep stairway that led to the front lobby. I passed two huge posters of Indian men seated in lotus position, one on a tiger skin. (Much later I would learn that this was Bikram Choudhury, the founder of this yoga. The other was another famous yogi, Paramahansa Yogananda.) Rounding the corner and going through another glass door, I was greeted at the front desk by a woman dressed in a sports bra and black short shorts. She seemed half naked.

As I signed a release form and paid for the class, a constant wave of people came through the door behind me, making it hard to hear what the woman at the desk was telling me.

"It's 105 degrees in the room and forty percent humidity," she said, raising her voice over the thunderous stomping of feet on the stairway and the growing chatter of the students sitting in the lobby. "Be good to yourself. Take a seat if you feel overwhelmed. Stay in the room. The instructor will tell you when to take water. Hold off until then. Any questions?"

7

I shook my head. I slipped off my shoes and put them on a rack in the lobby, copying the students swirling around me, and walked barefoot down the hallway to the ladies' changing room. Stuffing my bag in a row of cubbies in the cramped space of the changing room, I took my mat, beach towel and water bottle and pulled open the door to what the woman had called "The Hot Room."

Whatever ideas I had about what this yoga class would be quickly melted away even as I took my first steps into the room. I expected the space to be heated, but I didn't expect it to be 105 degrees before class had even begun. (I expected it to be like the commercials and magazines I had seen with people doing yoga poses, but with a little more sweat. I expected it to be a nice easy workout. A good stretch.) Nothing could have prepared me for the wall of heat that assaulted my body as I unrolled the mat and placed the beach towel over it. The air had a salty tang to it, paired with a tangible humidity that was already making me break a light sweat. I felt like I needed gills to breathe.

Other students quietly came in and placed their mats down. Some stayed and lay down as if tanning at the beach, while others did some light stretching. Most went back out the door and took a seat in the lobby as they waited for class to begin. I sat on top of my mat and towel and tried to look like I belonged.

Mirrors lined every inch of the room except for the back wall, and fluorescent lights hung from the ceiling, ready to shine down on the students. I felt intimidated and exposed as the newbie I was when I caught my reflection in the mirror and realized I had more clothes on than anybody else in the room. Men wore swim trunks with no shirts, and woman wore sports bras and capris, or tank tops and short shorts, or even more exposing a sports bra and short shorts like the woman at the front desk. There was even a woman at the front of the room wearing bikini bottoms instead of shorts. My tank top and capris looked out of place, as though I had worn a winter jacket to a summer barbecue.

The conversations and noise from the lobby quieted down until I was surrounded by a promising silence. A shifting of bodies taking their places made me look around with anticipation, and a flicker of the lights turning on signaled the entrance of the teacher. Young and attractive, he quietly demanded attention as he took his place on the podium at the front. He looked around at the people on their mats and asked if there were any first-time students in class that evening. I meekly raised my hand from my spot in the back row. I was the only newcomer that night. He nodded, threw a reassuring smile my way, and we began.

He told us to bring our feet together and interlace our fingers, placing our hands underneath our chins for a breathing exercise. In unison, the students that surrounded me then began to lift their elbows up to the ceiling so that their forearms were on either side of their faces. Then, on the instructor's cue, they all tipped their heads back, opened up their mouths and collectively made a raucous, windy "hah" noise as they brought their elbows together to touch in front of them. At first, I had no idea what was happening. It took me a few repetitions and watching a woman in the front row to understand the flow of this exercise. I tried to get the correct form so that my movements matched those of the students reflected back to me in the mirrors. The noise of the air rushing from my lungs, and those of the students on either side of me, made me want to giggle and cry at the same time. It seemed ridiculous and odd, but also familiar, reminding me of a breathing exercise my voice teacher used to start our lessons with when I was in the fifth grade. After two sets of ten repetitions my shoulders were achy, and I was already beading with sweat on my upper lip and forehead.

Then came the instructions for Half Moon Pose, the first posture in the class. I brought my arms over my head, once again interlacing my fingers but then adjusting the grip to match that of the students around me with the index fingers released to point up to the ceiling. I bent my upper body over to the right and tried to hold onto the pose as the instructor continued to talk, describing what we should be doing and what the best form would be. At this point, I was already regretting the clothes I had chosen. The cool and loose capris I often used as cover-ups after dance class (that earlier had looked like what I thought people wore to yoga) were already clinging to my legs in a most unattractive way as they sopped up each drop of sweat. I tried to ignore it as I came out of the posture and then bent over to the left, pushing my feet down into the mat to avoid falling over. As we went into a forward bend a few moments later, I pulled the legs of the capris down and away from my calf muscles, but I knew it was pointless—they were going to stick to my legs no matter what I did.

I continued to follow along with the rest of the class and move from posture to posture. Some of the movements were familiar, my body easily performing what was asked of it. Others, like Eagle Pose, boggled my mind as I watched the row of students in front of me gracefully cross one leg over the other and wrap their foot around the standing leg to create a twisted look. Their arms were mirroring the same action as one arm curled under the other and continued to twist together until the hands touched palm to palm.

"How are they doing that?" I thought as I hopped from side to side and tried to get my foot to hook behind my standing leg while weaving my arms together, elbows stacked and palms touching with my fingers interlaced into one large fist. My body wobbled and bobbled in the mirrors as I fought to find any kind of balance. On the second set, I decided just to blend in and be as still as possible as I could see that my movement was catching the attention of the woman in front of me. She was no longer watching herself in the front mirror but was instead staring at me with an amused smile. I crossed my arms into position, but didn't try to hook my foot and just waited for it to be over.

"Party time!" the instructor boomed over the microphone, and with that everyone leaned over, grabbed up water bottles and took a sip. I followed suit, gulping down the once icy but now lukewarm water I had brought into the room with me.

All too quickly, we moved onto the next set of postures. In what the instructor called Standing Bow Pulling Pose I felt a wave of relief that this was something I could accomplish. Grabbing my ankle with one hand, I stood on one leg and raised my opposite arm over my head. Then I followed the instructions to bring my body down while kicking and stretching to eventually create a standing split. Finally, something I understood! When I felt the teacher staring in my direction, I looked over his way.

"Dancer?" he asked.

I nodded and smiled, proud of what I was accomplishing as my heart rate rose and my face grew to a cherry red in the mirror with each minute ticking away in the hot room.

Toe Stand, the instructor promised, was the last standing posture of the class. I listened to the words and continued to watch the students around me as I made my first attempt. Standing on my left leg with my right foot placed on my left thigh, I bent forward at the hips to put my hands on the ground, and then bent my left knee to bring my hips to hover over my left heel. "How did I get down here and how am I going to get back out?" my mind questioned, surprised to find myself in this pretzel-shaped position, as my eyes darted around me for the answer.

"Good work back there," the instructor threw my way, and I smiled as sweat dripped into my eyes while I tried not to fall over.

Somehow, I made it out of Toe Stand without too much trouble, and then we all lay down on our mats in Savasana. I listened to the thump of my heart beating and wondered why I couldn't feel the air moving around me. It seemed as if there were no air at all. It was so hot. And stagnant. And impossible. Class had to be over soon. We had to be close to hitting the ninety-minute mark, right?

Actually, we were only about halfway there. We did a quick sit-up in which everyone around me made a loud noise with their breathing I didn't entirely understand and then turned over onto our stomachs.

"Spine Strengthening Series," the teacher said. "Cobra Pose."

As I placed my hands underneath my shoulders as instructed, I thought I knew what to expect. I had seen the cover of *Yoga Journal*. All I had to do was push my hands into the floor and lift my upper body up while keeping my legs straight and flat on the floor. When were told to lift up though, I realized quickly this was not what I had thought. The students surrounding me had stayed closer to the ground, their bent elbows on each side them, while I had launched my upper body into the air, elbows straight. I tried awkwardly to recover and lower down to the same level as the rest of the class.

I didn't understand the next posture, Locust Pose, at all. I put my arms underneath my body with my palms facing the floor as directed, but the position seemed wildly uncomfortable and a little painful.

"Put your mouth to the floor like you're kissing the towel," the instructor commanded. Reluctantly, I did as I was told, getting a close-up look at my sweat-soaked beach towel and trying not to get grossed out. Then we were instructed to lift both legs in the air.

"Sure," I thought, "Like that is even possible."

My legs didn't move at all. They were anchored to the floor. I gave up trying to get them to move and came out of the posture early to see that the older gentleman on the mat next to me was able to get both his legs up into the air at an impressive angle.

"Okay, maybe someday," I reassured myself, "but not tonight."

By the end of class I felt wrung out. If there had been any toxins in my body, they were long gone. I felt clean and beautifully tired, but in an unexplainably energetic way. I lay on my mat in the final Savasana, or Corpse Pose, for the required two minutes the teacher had encouraged at the end of class. Then I rolled up my mat and walked out of the hot room to be greeted by a blissful rush of cool air. I felt like I was gliding as I walked back to the changing room. Peeling off my clothes, which were now heavy with sweat and seemed to weigh about three pounds, I changed into the outfit I had packed to get me home.

At my car, I spread a towel on my seat in the hopes it would soak up the sweat that seemed, to my fascination, to continue to pour out of me. How was it possible I was still sweating?

The strange clean-sweaty-tired-energetic feeling was still with me when I got home about fifteen minutes later.

"Where were you?" Jeffrey asked, "Dance class?"

"No, I told you this morning I was thinking of taking that hot yoga class."

"How was it? Hot? Your face it beat red, Babe."

"It was… a challenge," I replied grinning. "I hope I can find the time to go back. I want to do that again. It was hard and ridiculous and fun to do something that had nothing to do with auditioning."

Later that night I climbed into bed to enjoy the first best sleep of my life. My arms and legs were heavy from the work they had been put through as they lifted, contracted and stretched in the heat. As I drifted off to sleep I sifted through everything I had coming up in the weeks ahead, looking for a spot for a return visit on my schedule. "I can go back in two weeks," I thought and smiled.

***

I found pockets of time here and there over the next year to get back to the studio. I'd rush home from work, change into a tank top and short shorts and make it to the studio in time for the 5:30 p.m. class at least once a month. Sometimes I would have a morning audition scheduled that required me to take time away from my temp job, and then I took the opportunity to sneak in an early morning class. Afterwards, I'd drive downtown or hop on the train and then sit for a few hours in the inevitable line of actors before it was my turn to sing my favorite sixteen bars of music or recite the monologue that best fit the character I was hoping to play. I always felt better after class, less anxious and more centered. During class I still wasn't sure why I liked it. It was still overwhelmingly hot, and I was far away from being able to accomplish some of the goals of each posture, but afterwards I felt the best I had in weeks.

Jeffrey soon grew curious about the class. He was coming off of a full year of running several half-marathons and marathons in quick succession. After months of waking up before sunrise to train and rack up his miles before heading off to school, Jeffrey was now officially injured. He was experiencing extreme pain in his legs and feet, and had gone from athletic and active to having regular appointments with a physical therapist and prescribed orthotics. He was thirty-two.

Needing to find some kind of physical activity he could do without putting too much stress on his joints, he asked - and I found myself answering—question after question about the Bikram Yoga: "So how hot is it exactly?" "Can you show me what some of the postures look like?" "How long is the class again?" "Do you have to stay for the whole thing?"

After weeks of this, I told him I had had enough of the questions and that he needed to put on swim trunks or running shorts and just come along with me. We made a date to attend class that night.

I had some apprehension taking him with me. This would be the first time I had brought anyone to the studio and I had seen, at the handful of classes that I had taken, how some people had reacted negatively to the lights, mirrors, heat, and structure of the class - sometimes even leaving the room, looking white lipped and as if they were going to faint or puke any minute. Jeffrey is also a known perfectionist, and I often joke with him about how he's either all-in or all-out. This yoga class would be his one shot at the practice. Either he would like it or hate it. If he hated it, the chances were slim that he would try it again.

On our way to the studio I explained to him the rules of the class. "Do not talk to me in the hot room. There's no talking once class begins, and it can be embarrassing if the teacher asks you to remain quiet. And please try not to leave. Once it starts you're in there for ninety-minutes if you like it or not."

Unrolling our mats in the hot room, I felt a surge of anxiety. I seemed to be more nervous for his first class than I had been for my own. We placed his mat a few feet behind mine, so I could visually help him out when he needed it, and then we went out to the lobby to wait for class to begin.

As the teacher checked in the last students and locked the door, we walked back into the hot room and took our places on our mats. The lights flickered on, and the boom of the instructor's voice over the microphone rang through the humid, hot air.

With the completion of each posture, I was surprised at how easily Jeffrey handled the class. Dripping and red faced like the rest of us, he seemed fine with the heat, the mirrors, and the constant chatter of the instructor. In the standing postures I slowly demonstrated the grips so he could follow along, and in Locust Pose I showed him how to flip his hands so his palms were facing the mat instead of grabbing his thighs. At the end of class we lay in Savasana and, as we rolled our heads towards each other, we caught each other's eyes and smiled. I knew then he would be back.

And as expected, since Jeffrey enjoyed the intensity of the class, he was all-in. He stopped going to his physical therapy sessions and soon had us at the yoga studio three times a week, waking me up early on Saturday and Sunday mornings for weekend sessions in the hot room. Within a few months, this turned into five times a week, and then we found ourselves standing on our mats in the hot room almost every day.

His enthusiasm for the practice made me want to make my own practice a priority, and I started scheduling my music and acting lessons and classes only once or twice a week instead of every single night so that I could get to the studio.

About a year into his practice, Jeffrey touched his toes with straight legs for the first time in his entire life and no longer complained about his running injuries, which seemed to have dissipated. I was able to hook my foot in Eagle Pose and had developed an impressive back bend. We were both amazed at how our bodies were opening up and changing for the better.

End of the day talks now consisted of how to get deeper into a posture, what correction we heard at class that night, and which teachers we liked the best. We read the books written by Bikram Choudhury, the man who developed the yoga we had become devoted to, in order to learn even more when we were at home and away from the studio. We invested in hot yoga mats made to absorb the seeming gallons of sweat coming off of us during class and even clingy, teeny hot yoga clothes. The practice seemed to have woven its way into every fiber of our life. We were yogis.

A Yoga Teacher's Letter to Her First-Time Student

From the Blog: January 6, 2016

Dear First Timer:

You don't even realize how amazing you were throughout your first class! You stayed in that hot, sticky, drippy room the entire time. You followed instructions. You took a seat when you needed one. You even found stillness during Savasana.

I know you are doubting these words right now. I know that you looked at the folks in the front row and had the thought, "That will never be me. They must have been born with freakish flexibility or godly strength." But I'm here to tell you that they started the same way you did, following along, trying their best, and wondering how they had found themselves in this crazy yoga class. The only thing they did that others sometimes do not, is come back. And not just a couple of times, but again and again and again as they looked for a way to master the class, to master their bodies, their minds, and their breath. To master their lives.

I wish that for you. That you come back. That you try again. You might feel resistance to this practice. You might find an excuse why it isn't for you. It was too hot. The teacher was too loud, her voice booming through the microphone, so that you could not even pretend not to hear her. And at times she even called out your name to encourage or correct you, and you wished with every loud beat of your heart pounding in your ears that she would simply leave you alone. It was too bright and the mirrors were too much, as you watched your face turn an alarming shade of red. You might even have a headache tonight (as your body urges you to drink more water and eat better food) after you dripped with what seemed like buckets of sweat throughout the class.

I hear you. Yoga is not easy. It is a challenge. Taking up a regular yoga practice is one of the bravest things you can do in life. It means you are willing to become better than you are today. It means you are ready to take responsibility for your own life's story and face yourself on the soul level for ninety or sixty minutes, day after day, to discover where you are locked up, both physically and mentally, in order to free yourself from past injury and emotional turmoil. It is more than a workout. It is a work in.

I hope I see you in my class again. For me, there's nothing better than sharing this yoga, and I want to share it with you. I look forward to the day you look in the mirrors and smile at what you see or maybe even pull your mat up to the front row, so you can really get a good look at you and your practice and where you are in that moment. For someday, if you stick with it, you will find your own strength and your own flexibility, in *and* out of the studio and you, my friend, will shine.

Sincerely,
Your Yoga Teacher

CHAPTER TWO

THE BEST FOOD IS NO FOOD?

Tall is a way of being in my family. My father stands at an even six feet and is considered short compared to his three brothers, who all surpass him in height by at least three or four inches. One of my uncles stands over six and a half feet tall. My mom was the tallest woman in her family (at five-foot-six) - until my sister and I came along, that is. Once I got my growth spurt at age twelve I passed her. There was no way around it: I was going to be tall.

And tall is okay, but I was also round. Clothes never fit me right. Shopping for back-to-school clothes was the worst, as my mom would help me tug on what seemed like an endless series of pants and then groan as each pair failed to fit. Jeans at that time weren't made for an eight-year-old who actually had a butt and a tummy, so I always walked out of the store with corduroys in five different colors.

At school I craved the attention that the petite girls often received, as teachers, parents and fellow students would admire their cuteness, while I would best be described as a "big" girl, or politely described as "statuesque." At night I would lie in bed looking down the length of my body. I would scan the top of my pink pajamas, where my belly with its squishy baby fat poked through, and my legs, stretching out beyond imagination, with thighs that seemed twice the size of the other girls' in my third grade class. This body did not feel like it belonged to me. If it did, it should look like I expected it to look. It was too much somehow. I took up too much space.

My older sister, Tara, was even taller than I was and also seemed uncomfortable about it, slouching to appear shorter for most of her childhood. There was a distinct difference between our looks, though, as she had the sought-after willowy frame popular among super models and ballet dancers. Tara could eat a pound of gummy bears in one sitting and not gain an ounce. People would stop her at the mall and ask if she modeled, telling her she should as she shook her head and smiled at the compliment.

I, on the other hand, learned at an early age to count calories and manage my intake of food. With each passing year I grew and continued to tower over the other kids in my class. Moving into the awkwardness of puberty, the connection to my body seemed to get worse. Now, there were boobs and a belly *and* my overly large thighs. In the summer before sixth grade, there was a shift when I grew another inch and the belly went away, but I felt like it was still

24

there. I was a straight-A student at the top of my class, and I felt like I could control anything and be good at anything. I felt I had no limits - except my body.

With the pressure to be noticed by the boys in my middle school I made a pact with my girlfriend, Meghan, to lose weight so we could have the slimmer bodies we both wanted.

"Let's do this together," I said to her one day when we were both complaining about not being skinny enough.

The pact was simple: no food. I would go to her house every morning before the school bus came, and we would pour out a small glass of orange juice, planning on having that as our only nourishment for the entire day. At lunchtime, we would distract ourselves by studying or doing homework. We would sit on the floor with our backs against the row of lockers that lined the cafeteria and try to ignore the boisterous throng of kids at the tables in front of us as they feasted on potato chips and Whatchamacallit Bars they had microwaved to a gooey perfection. At dinner with my family, I became talented at pushing food around my plate, feeding scraps to our dog, Biscuits, and taking a few bites before heading off to read or practice piano. Most days no one seemed to notice I wasn't eating. On the days they did, I would begrudgingly finish my dinner, knowing I could burn off the calories later.

Exercise became my obsession. If I didn't have to stay after school for choir or basketball practice, I would be down in the basement with a workout tape, lunging and crunching in time with the body-perfect woman on the screen who smiled and cheered me on through each task. My younger brother, Michael, would come down and nag me to finish so he could play Mario Brothers. I would yell at him to get out as I struggled through my third round of crunches that promised six pack abs. My mom was proud of me for working out and taking care of myself, and would shoo Michael away, telling him he could have the basement when I was finished.

When the weather was good, I would go out on a two- or three-mile run, dressed in an oversized running jacket that had been my dad's, grasping my yellow Sony Walkman in my right hand and charging through the neighborhood. I enjoyed the freedom that running gave me. It made me feel powerful and in control. But no matter how many miles I would rack up each week, I would look in the mirror and still see big, **big**, **BIG**.

By the time I was a freshman in high school I had developed a full-on eating disorder. Meghan, a year ahead of me, had long given up our pact as she went on to high school without me, but we still waved at each other as we passed in the hallways. She wasn't as driven as I was to stay fit and lose weight, and she seemed to have found her own sense of self with her new circle of friends. She had gotten involved in the school newspaper and French Club, while I was on the other side of the building, singing my heart out or working on a piece of choreography for the competitive show choir that took up every moment of my time. Dreams of Broadway echoed in every corner of my mind. I was working hard at developing a very good voice and clean, polished steps. On top of those, if I became skinny enough and beautiful enough, I could make it. I knew I could.

Busy going from rehearsal to rehearsal, I rarely hung out at home. I appeared to be a happy, singing, dancing, performing kid. On the outside I brimmed with confidence, but on the inside, I was a world-class bully.

I ate next to nothing and soon began purchasing and taking laxatives and water pills, having gotten the idea from an *ABC Afterschool Special* about a girl who developed an eating disorder to cope with her problems. The story was supposed to deter girls from heading down this path, but for me it was instructional. I would never take it as far as that girl in the show. I wasn't going to die from this. She was obviously crazy and I was not. I was in control. I would be smart about it. I just had to get to the point where I felt light on my feet and beautiful under the stage lights and get compliments like, "Wow, you look great! Have you lost weight?"

Life was a balancing act. I couldn't always starve myself and still do what I needed to do. There were times I had to eat more, like after a long rehearsal, as my body would announce its need for food, giving me a pounding headache and making me feel light headed. I had to stay sharp to pick up the steps in choreography sessions, memorize the music for the next rehearsal, nail my piano lesson, ace the math test, write the essay for my lit class, and rise to the top of my class.

It was all about performing. It was all about being perfect. And then I fell in love.

Dion was a senior and in choir, but he was also on the football team and played the trumpet in the band and was funny and smart.

He was adorable. Sitting in the bleachers at a football game in the fall of my junior year, I blushed uncontrollably when our eyes met as he looked up at the crowd from the field, smiled, and waved in my direction. We had been paired together a few times in show choir rehearsal to learn the steps of the choreography, and we found that we enjoyed working together, laughing when we made the wrong move, yet working during our breaks to get it just right.

I had gone out on a few dates by that point, but nothing special: a few guys from choir, a very attractive boy in my gym class (who seemed absolutely dreamy until he revealed that he hated to read and only enjoyed heavy metal bands), a boy I'd been good friends with all through elementary and middle school (we realized were just great friends).

Dion was different. We gravitated towards each other for the entire fall semester, stopping to chat in the hallway between classes, working next to each other at a Music Boosters fundraising event, and inviting each other out in large groups of friends to the movies or to hang out at the local Denny's with the other kids from school.

It wasn't until February that we went on an actual date. One day in the choir room after class I was looking through my music as all the other kids filtered out towards their ride home or to their afterschool activity, and Dion took a seat next to me. He asked if I'd like to go to the movies that weekend. My heartbeat quickened in my chest as I said yes and we made plans for that Saturday night.

From that moment on we were inseparable, and I discovered it wasn't as easy to keep going with my plan for perfection as it had been when I was single. Dating with an eating disorder is tough work. Popcorn at the movies? Let's go out to eat? It only took a few dates until he gently asked if I had a problem.

Sitting in his car in my driveway after our third date, Dion cut the ignition and shifted in his seat to turn his body toward mine.

"We need to talk," he said with a worried frown. I thought he was about to break up with me, but then he said, "Don't you eat? I'm starting to notice you hardly eat anything at all. What's going on?"

Tears filled my eyes. I felt humiliated at being caught and relieved at the same time that someone had finally noticed.

He leaned toward me and put his arms around my shoulders, looking deeply in to my eyes. I looked away.

"Please, look at me. I don't mean to upset you, but what you're doing is dangerous."

After a few deep breaths, I met his eyes, feeling defeated in so many ways. "Please, don't tell anyone," I pleaded. "I can stop."

"Listen, I really like you and I want to keep seeing you, but I can't do that if you're going to continue to starve yourself. You don't need to do that stuff. You're already beautiful," he said and I melted.

So that night, I resolved to stop. If Dion had noticed my eating disorder, than maybe I had gone too far. I didn't want to disappoint anyone, especially my parents. If they found out, I felt like they wouldn't understand. And I knew Dion would tell them if I continued.

I discovered I couldn't just will my eating habits away so easily. I still watched my food intake, counted every calorie and scrutinized each inch of my body in the wall of rehearsal mirrors at the dance studio and in the choir room. I began to eat regularly, but I did it to make Dion happy, to show him I was fine, that there was nothing to worry about, instead of stopping for myself. Big mistake.

Our relationship lasted a total of eight months. We dated through the spring, sitting next to each other as we rode on the coach buses to show choir competitions throughout the Midwest, preparing for the final choir concert and the end of the school year. I watched Dion get his diploma as he walked across the stage among four hundred other graduates, and then it was time to enjoy the summer months together.

Dion and I wanted to make as many memories as possible before he left for college in the fall. We took trips to the Michigan Dunes and enjoyed walking along the beach along Lake Michigan, stopping to simply sit in the sand and talk. We went to Six Flags and waited in long lines to feel the rush of adrenaline as we plunged towards the earth on the rollercoasters, turning, up, down, and around and then laughing at the fun of it. Dion got a group of friends together for a weekend camping trip, sharing stories around the fire and hiking through the woods. My hand was always in his. If we weren't together, we were on the phone or planning to get together soon, always finding another movie we could go to or restaurant we wanted to try.

In the fall, it seemed strange to go back to school without him. We talked on the phone every day at first. He came home often, and we pretended that nothing had changed. But it had. Dion was meeting new people and having new experiences, and I couldn't relate to what was going on at the time. I took a trip one weekend to visit him at college and tried not to be awkward around his roommate and at the party we went to on Saturday night. But I felt so young compared to everyone else - the high school girlfriend.

At the end of October, Dion came home for another visit. We went out to eat, enjoyed catching up with each other, and held hands the entire time. When he dropped me off at home late that night and walked me to the door, he asked if we could sit on the porch swing for a while. Then he carefully explained that we needed to break up, avoiding my eyes as he said the words that would end everything. He explained that his grades were suffering, and his parents were getting upset that he was coming home so much when he should be focused on his college work.

I couldn't believe what I was hearing. We had just had a great night together. How was this happening? Tears rolled down my cheeks and I started to sob.

"Please don't cry. I still love you, but I have to be at school. This just doesn't work anymore."

I cried on and off for weeks. I packed all of the gifts he had given me and all the tokens of our time together. I put them into a black trash bag and stored it away in the crawlspace in our garage. I was heartbroken.

And as the weeks passed, a thought snaked its way into my mind: if I had been skinnier and if I had been prettier, maybe he would have stayed.

I fell right back the spiral of my eating disorder during my senior year. I ran every day, farther and farther. Two miles turned into an average of six. No breakfast, I didn't need it. Mashed potatoes (no gravy) from the school cafeteria for lunch. I went back to nibbling at dinner and pushing the food around my plate until everyone was done and I could leave the table. If I needed a snack, I would make air-popped popcorn. I popped laxatives and water pills. For the first time, I tried to force myself to vomit. I couldn't get the hang of it, so I only did it if I absolutely felt I had too much to eat.

Pounds dropped off. I had gone down a size in my jeans and luxuriated in shopping for new ones admiring the number six on the tag. My show choir competition dress floated around my frame instead of hugging my torso in its fitted styling. All my hard work was paying off. I received accolades from my girlfriends and even from a dance teacher I worked with. I loved the attention and wanted more of it.

All of this came to a tipping point at the Music Booster's Spring Fashion Show Fundraiser. I was one of the student models set to strut the runway while ladies lunched on banquet food and admired the clothes from local retailers, all in the name of supporting music in my school. My mom had purchased tickets so that both of my sisters and my grandma could attend and enjoy the afternoon.

After the show I changed my clothes in what would be considered the backstage area for the event, and then went to meet my mom in the lobby. She was standing at the edge of the hallway with Tara. My younger sister, Jenny, and my grandma were still in the banquet hall, claiming the raffle prize my grandma had won at the end of the event.

My mom is beautiful. She keeps her hair cut short in a caramel-blond color that offsets her deep blue eyes. Dainty and feminine, she has womanly curves and a kind smile that is attractive to everyone around her. She works hard for her physique. First, she was into aerobics, taking class almost every day at her health club, and then she became a personal trainer. She also runs marathons a couple of times a year. My mom is strong and athletic and most of all believes in me. When no one else thought I had any singing talent, my mom walked me into the bathroom and told me to belt it out and listen to what I heard so that I could make it better. She always made me feel like I could do anything and be anyone.

But this day, she seemed angry. Her jaw was tense, and I could see in her eyes that something was wrong.

"How was lunch?" I asked, hoping I was misreading the energy pulsing off her body.

"We need to talk," she replied. "Tara found these in your dresser drawer this morning. What are doing with these?"

Her eyes were now wide and imploring as she held out a plastic-and-foil-wrapped sheet of laxatives.

My heart raced and my face suddenly felt hot as tears welled in my eyes. Humiliated, yet aware of my surroundings, as the lobby filled with parents and peers from my school, I wiped the tears away and mumbled, "I'm just trying to lose some weight."

Mom furrowed her brow and cocked her head to force me to meet her eyes.

"This is not the way to do it. You know better than this. We'll talk about this at home."

The drive home seemed interminable. There was no way out of this. My mom was disappointed, which meant my dad was disappointed, which meant this was the worst possible outcome. I had failed.

After a long, uncomfortable discussion in which I lied about how long this had been going on and promised to stop immediately, I apologized to my mom, feeling comforted as she gave me a long hug.

"You've got it all, Tori. You have so much confidence. You're smart and talented. Don't blow it."

It seemed like she was talking about someone else. The voice in my head told me I could always be more. Smarter. More talented. Skinnier. But in that moment her words helped.

I could do this the right way. I could stop.

And I did.

And then I didn't.

MAT TO MAT CHAT

CLAUDIA

Like many women, Claudia's life involved taking care of others. She was a teacher, a single mother, a sister, a daughter. With all that caregiving, there was one person she was overlooking. What Claudia had to learn was how to take care of herself. Her yoga story begins with an ending.

"My dad died in my arms," she says. "It was one of my greatest heartbreaks. I buried him on my birthday. I took care of him for a long time. It was a slow, slow death. He was a vibrant person, but towards the end he couldn't even walk up the stairs."

Not long after her father's death, Claudia was looking for holistic alternatives to high blood pressure for her sister Patti. She discovered countless articles that touted Bikram Yoga as a great way to counteract high blood pressure, so she found a local studio, grabbed her sister, and got to class.

They sweated their way through their first class, giggling at the pure craziness of the practice. "Are you kidding me?" they whispered to each other in disbelief as the teacher tried to keep them focused and on task from the podium.

After that first class, Claudia recalls feeling "like I had a hangover for days, as if I had been drinking forever," but that didn't stop her from signing up for a membership. At first, she attended sporadically. Eventually, tired of wasting money on something she wasn't using, she stopped at the front desk after an evening class to cancel her membership. The studio owner steered Claudia away from quitting. She offered both Claudia and Patti a work-trade (Karma Yoga) position, in which they would do light cleaning at the studio each week in exchange for free classes.

Claudia was relieved that this arrangement could keep Patti involved at the studio and showing up to class. But Claudia found herself still resistant to the yoga; she would do the cleaning and then leave, rarely setting foot in the hot room for her own practice.

"I didn't even like to look at myself. I wish someone told me from the beginning to look at yourself, keep your feet together, and stand up straight. I hated being in the hot room because I struggled," she admits.

Around this time she met a man and began a relationship. Claudia hadn't dated in a long time. The man was funny and attractive, but from the beginning she noticed he seemed to drink too much.

Finding herself in the hot room one night for practice, she realized that when she thought about this new relationship, in her gut she knew it wasn't good for her.

"Every day I would wake up with knots in my stomach and think, 'I've got to get out of this,' but I couldn't. I think I was afraid of hurting his feelings or something stupid like that."

And then the unthinkable happened. One evening out, while Claudia was driving, they got into an argument. With little warning he lost his temper and hit her. It only took one moment of violence for Claudia to know she was done. She never spoke to him again.

"That moment was the thing that helped me get out of a situation I knew I needed to leave behind. I started thinking, 'What am I doing with my life that I'm attracting this garbage?' From there, I knew I had to step back and truly look at a lot of things. The way I was projecting myself, the way I interacted with others, my grieving process over my dad's death, my parenting, my job as a teacher. Everything."

Deciding she needed to take some time putting herself first to cleanse herself of this toxic relationship, Claudia began a Sixty-Day Challenge - sixty classes in sixty days without missing a single day. During this time, she found she was able to get clear about what she wanted for her life.

"Yoga was able to help put in perspective what is valuable to me. I used to work crazy hours as an ESL teacher and be stressed out all of the time. I learned that some things in life are not worth the energy to get worked up about."

In an effort to gain clarity, Claudia decided to write down exactly what she wanted in a partner. She felt she needed to be clear about what was acceptable and what was not, so that she would never be stuck in a similar relationship.

Not long after she had completed her challenge, she met her brother's friend, Jay. Jay's an ironworker, whose work often involves traveling to projects. He was living in Tennessee at the time, forcing them to take things slowly in their new relationship, as Claudia had no desire to move away from family and friends.

Early in their relationship, Claudia started bringing Jay to yoga when he was in town. He was a champion in the hot room, sticking it out, asking questions after class, and supporting Claudia's love for the yoga. He was a keeper. He was everything she had put on her ideal partner list when she was looking for clarity, when she started to reach for the life she deserves. She had found a great guy, a true partner, and a man who loved and cared not only for her, but for her daughter as well. Jay became her husband.

One of my favorite interactions with Claudia was when I asked her to demonstrate Locust Pose for the rest of the students in class. She looked at me, horrified at the request.

"Claudia, it's a gorgeous pose. I *wish* I had your Locust. Get your arms underneath you and let's show it off!" I pleaded.

She rolled her eyes, smiled, and then got into position, raising her legs in the air with ease as she pushed her arms down into the floor. Then, as she slowly came out of the posture, the whole class applauded her achievement, inspired to try and lift their legs high off the floor.

Claudia recognizes the breadth of the achievements that yoga has helped her bring about and the changes she has seen.

"I'm proud of the investment I've taken with my practice— getting the good water bottles and clothes, reading the books, taking the posture clinics. It means I'm serious about it and I've never had anything like that before. This is the only physical activity I love. I'm taller - I've grown an inch - I'm now five-foot three. I'm finally okay with my body. I'm not easily distracted or anxious," she explains. And it's not just her. "My sister, Patti is off of her blood pressure medication completely. Most of all, I can't believe the amazing people I've met. I never knew anyone around town and now I've met people that I consider my friends."

She also understands that the changes had to come when she was ready for them.

"It took many classes to get where I am today. I'm approaching my 400th class in four years. It's cool to compare where I began to where I am now in my practice and in my life. When I think about it, I feel like that quote from Rumi, 'The wound is where the light enters you.' Yoga helped me find my light."

CHAPTER THREE

ACTING, MARRIAGE & MIRACLES

Life went on. The end of my senior year came and went. I performed for the last time with my show choir, I graduated, and I nervously looked towards the future. In college, I would not be donning sequins and chiffon when I performed. I would not be memorizing the latest pop hit or Broadway show tune. I would be majoring in vocal performance, working on classical music, arias, and developing techniques that would help me maintain my voice for a long career. Actually, I would be double majoring, also getting a degree in music education, as my dad said that the only job I could get with a vocal performance degree would be at a fast-food joint, and he wanted me to have a back-up plan.

Although I was nervous, I was also excited, because college was my chance for me to reinvent myself. Having graduated with kids that I had known since elementary school, this was a chance for me to start fresh, surrounded by new people. This was a chance for me to have always appeared perfect and skinny to those I would meet. That summer I worked out more than before. I ran longer. I ate less. I caved and bought laxatives and water pills, but hid them somewhere new. I was careful to be discreet, and no one noticed that I might be falling back into old patterns. They trusted me when I said I could stop.

In the fall of 1995 I arrived at Illinois State University ready (I thought) for the next chapter in my life. I hadn't seen or heard from Dion in months and felt healed of my broken heart and ready for something new. My dorm was located almost a mile away from the quad, which led to endless complaints from most of the students placed there, but I liked it. It was built-in exercise.

My roommate, Kelly, was the exact opposite of me, but for some reason it seemed to work. Kelly was a business major. She didn't seem overly excited about it or passionate about it like I was about music and singing. She was short (five-foot-one) and curvy with sparkling eyes and chestnut brown hair. She was relaxed in the places I was keyed up and stressed. We complimented each other well and seemed to get along naturally.

As a music major, my schedule was locked in from the beginning. While other freshman could plow through their general education classes, I was in music theory, group piano, voice lessons, choir, and music education lab classes, with time for only two general education classes squeezed in each semester. There was a pressure of a different kind too, as I had to continue to perform at my best in every class, so I could move on to the next level each semester. If I failed a class in the program, that class wouldn't come around again until the next year, leaving me far behind my peers.

The college experience wasn't all about grades and classes though. On the first day of college choir a very cute, kind of odd (in an alluring way) upperclassman took the seat next to me and began flirting outrageously with me. His head was shaved bald, which was eccentric in 1995, but it suited him, making his brown eyes pop. As the class sang I enjoyed his confidence and the way his smooth tenor voice rang out into the space.

"I didn't catch your name," I said after rehearsal had finished.

"Jeffrey," he replied and winked at me before picking up his backpack and strolling out of the room. There was something about him.

Within the first week I noticed Jeffrey seemed to be almost everywhere I went. He had a class in the same building I did in the mornings, he was in the same voice studio as I was, and he led the first choir lab class. He also seemed to always choose to sit close to me in choir and make some kind of small talk when it ended, before we went our separate ways. I would start my walk towards my dorm and he would go in the opposite direction towards the apartment he had at the edge of campus.

Unfortunately, during the first weeks of school, I also seemed to be getting sick constantly. First, I had a cold, then I spent a weekend with the flu. One week in there I felt okay, but then the stomach cramps started. They would get so bad I could only curl up in the fetal position and hope they would end soon. Something was wrong.

A month into college I went to Student Health Services, hoping to get some help. It hadn't crossed my mind that my stomach problems had anything to do with my eating disorder. When the doctor asked about my eating habits, peering down my throat and pressing gently in between my ribs to get an idea what was going on with my stomach, he didn't seem surprised at all when I told him I didn't eat.

"How long has this been going on?" he asked with genuine concern.

"On and off for years," I admitted, gulping as the feeling of shame overtook me and tears once again started stinging my eyes.

He didn't say much after that, just raised his eyebrows and pursed his lips, giving me some tips to stop the stomach cramps. Then he told me to take the elevator upstairs to the office for the university therapists and make an appointment.

"I'll call the receptionist right now and tell her to expect you," he instructed.

As I walked the mile and a half back to my dorm room through the chilled autumn gloom with a bag full of Pedialyte, antacids, and a slip for an appointment the following day with one of the therapists, I couldn't help but wonder how I had gotten into this mess. I was scared. My body was finally fighting back.

I started eating. I went to therapy each week. I cried and told my story to the young master's student that was functioning as my therapist. It helped to have someone that didn't know me listen and not judge me.

Jeffrey asked me out on a date a few weeks after my therapy started. He drove up to the front door of my dorm in his blue '76 Cutlass Oldsmobile. The engine (which he had rebuilt himself to make the car go insanely fast) roared as he stepped on the accelerator, hurtling us down the street. We went to Chili's for dinner. We talked for over two hours, enjoying chips and salsa, and I even ate a mushroom burger as we got to know each other amidst the chatter of the other diners.

"You must be feeling better," he smiled. "You didn't look too good a couple of weeks ago."

"Yeah, my stomach was acting up," I confessed, pausing to swallow and weigh my options of telling him what was going on. "I used to have an eating disorder."

The weight of the words hit me as I realized I had put it in the past tense.

"What? You didn't eat?" he asked.

"Pretty much. My stomach was bothering me because of that. I'm feeling much better now."

"You seem to be eating fine tonight," he said, smiling again.

After dinner, he took me to a local park a few miles from campus so we could continue talking as we walked down the marked trail. Stopping at a memorial statue at the edge of the park, he pulled me towards him and kissed me. It left me reeling. I was smitten.

Soon I was so involved at school and with Jeffrey that I felt I actually had conquered my eating disorder. I still exercised, lifting weights and lunging and jumping at five o'clock in the morning, with Kelly dead asleep in her bed. After classes, I'd hit the local running trail or get on a treadmill at the gym and run three or four miles.

After the fall semester was over, I gave up on the therapy. There seemed to be no point in rehashing the same story over and over again, and the therapist didn't seem to be giving me any tools to cope when I was feeling out of control. Plus, I wasn't feeling out of control or anxious as much. I had relaxed into a solid relationship with Jeffrey, made a great group of girlfriends at my dorm, and was busy keeping up with schoolwork. I was cured.

Two years into our relationship, I bought a pair of size ten jeans. Somehow, I had gotten comfortable, maybe *too* comfortable. I liked being the girl Jeffrey wanted me to be - healthy, happy, and able to sit down and chow on a great meal at a restaurant or chug beers with him at weekend parties.

But, in the middle of my sophomore year, Jeffrey graduated and took his first job, teaching choir in the Quad Cities. Two hours away. Going into my junior year, three long years without him on campus stretched before me, as I was in a five-year program. I worried that I had somehow recreated the same situation with Jeffrey that I had had with Dion. I was nervous our relationship would fall apart and that we wouldn't be able to make the distance work. With Jeffrey gone, there would be no one on campus wondering what I was up to and filling up my free time. Now I just had me. Again.

Without an anchor to keep me grounded and distracted from the thought of too fat, not good enough, my eating disorder slowly started up again. It wasn't a decision I made one day. I didn't say, "Today is the day I start to really dive back into my eating disorder." My obsession with food and exercise reappeared bit-by-bit, piece-by-piece until there was no denying that I was not cured of my eating disorder. I had simply stuffed it away some place safe until I needed it again.

I became obsessive about my exercise routine. Soon I was running at least six miles every morning before showering, sipping on some orange juice, and power walking across the quad to my eight o'clock class. Coming home after hours in a soundproof practice room, trying to get that Rossini aria just right for the end of the semester recital, I would reflexively pop in a workout tape and get in some more exercise before I went back to my studies. I ate, but not a lot. I recorded every calorie, carb, and fat gram in a notebook I kept with me at all times, proud when I was able to write less and less each day. I would look in the mirror and pinch at the skin on my hips or belly and try and imagine myself thinner.

I believed wholeheartedly that if I looked the way I dreamed of looking, I would be happy and could relax at last. What a lie! The thing is, when I look back at pictures from that time, I *did* look the way I wanted to look, but I couldn't see it for the life of me. All I could concentrate on was the reflection of the too big, too tall, too ugly, how-could-Jeffrey-ever-find-me-attractive mess that I saw in the mirror.

Jeffrey and I had our ups and downs during our first year apart. We saw each other most weekends during the school year, but even during visits both of us were busy as he prepared for his classes and I worked on finishing up my course work. The drive to and from the Quad Cities became second nature to me. Our time together was enough to keep me from letting my eating disorder completely take over, although I sometimes wondered whether it was too much to stay together, not wanting to get hurt as I had in the past.

Just before Christmas in 1998 at his school's holiday choir concert in front of all his students and their families, Jeffrey dramatically got down on one knee and asked me to marry him. Of course, I said yes. After that every weekend seemed packed with wedding planning. I was still juggling classes, student teaching, and trying to figure out what life would look like once I graduated. There was pressure, but I felt assured. Jeffrey and I were going to be married. We couldn't picture life without each other.

We were both into running at that point and had begun hitting the trails in the Quad Cities and on campus whenever we were together. I still wished I could be thinner. I would skip a meal here and there, but I felt I had everything under control. One week I would be incredibly strict with myself, exercising too much and eating next to nothing, and then the following week I would relax and eat.

In the spring of 2000 I graduated and in the fall Jeffrey and I married. Our plan was to stay in the Quad Cities for a few years (and then eventually move back to Chicago). I got a job as a singing waitress at the local professional theater. There were about ten of us on the floor at any time. We would serve the patrons of the theater and then before the show started, hop up on stage and perform for about fifteen minutes. It was great training. I had to think fast to be able to pour a cup of coffee and then jump on stage to sing a solo a moment later.

I would work a minimum of four shifts a week, catching time with Jeffrey on Saturday and Sunday mornings before driving to work. During the week I wouldn't see him until late at night when I returned home after the show. Rehearsals for each show were held on weekdays before our shifts.

The wait staff performed fifteen-minute shows that complemented whatever main stage show was playing. The shows were clever, created by the other waiters on staff who introduced me to new music and choreography each eight to ten-week period. When a new show was introduced, Jeffrey would come and cheer me on, happy that I was happy to be performing.

After I had performed in several of the wait staff shows, I got to be music director for one. Then I was then asked to choreograph some of the numbers, getting more involved each time as we worked to create the shows. Soon the producer of the theater took notice, and I landed my first paid acting gig in one of the children's shows, playing Rabbit in *Winnie the Pooh*. A few months later I played in the chorus of *Footloose* on the main stage.

Other work started to come. I booked two shows in Kansas, which led to being booked on a couple of shows in Arizona, which led to getting booked at a theater in downstate Illinois.

It was everything I had dreamed of as a child. I was being paid to sing and dance for a living. Most days I could hardly believe my luck even though I had worked so hard for this dream to come true. Once I was hired for a show it all seemed magical somehow. There were rehearsals and music and dancing and costumes to fill my days.

And this is when life got tricky. As my career took off theaters would fly me out and feed and house me for months on end at locations all over the country. I considered myself lucky if I was at home with Jeffrey for a month out of the year - and this was before iPhones, Skype, and the assumption that I would have Internet access at the drop of a hat.

I felt intense pressure all of the time to appear perfect—in looks and actions, finding the right mix of coming across as humble but bold, sweet yet sassy. No one wanted to hire a performer who created extra drama or had issues that would get in the way of good, consistent work. I knew of talented people who couldn't book a job because they had been difficult to work with or caused too much trouble, and people in this industry talk to each other constantly, so word gets around. If I had one major screw up, it could mean the end of my career.

I caved to the pressure. After years of thinking my eating disorder days were behind me, I welcomed back the abuse to my body and mind like opening the door to dearly missed friend. It crept back into my life little by little, but soon my eating disorder took over. And I wasn't the only one with a problem. In the theater I was surrounded by other women with the same food and body issues. The all-consuming pressure to appear perfect was overwhelming.

After three years on the road I was a wreck. I'd work out like a fiend, running five or six miles before I strapped on my four-inch character shoes and embarked an all-day rehearsal. I ate little and when I did, I wouldn't feel comfortable until I threw it up. Water pills were my best friend. I was insane, and I had very little respect for the body I had been given.

I closed myself off from my cast mates and kept everyone at arm's length, while at the same time craving their approval. If fellow actors talked behind my back or treated me with a snobbish disregard, I would act like their best friend and pay as much attention to them and shower them with as much love as possible. I trusted others' opinions of me more than I trusted my own gut and intuition. Instead of embracing my talents and sharing them, I ended up being embarrassed by the choices I would make at an audition or on stage. Then I'd cover up the embarrassment with a steely exterior I thought would be attractive to those making the casting and hiring choices.

I was a mess. The eating disorder let me feel in control of something when I couldn't control how others perceived me or how

I was cast - or not cast - in a show. I could control my food. I could control my exercise routine. But the control was an illusion, and I was miserable. This was markedly the lowest point of my life.

Staying over at my parents' house one night after yet another day of auditioning, I had finally broke down. I felt so empty, both emotionally and physically. Once the tears started, I couldn't stop them. I sat on the floor by the bed and rocked myself back and forth. I heard my own voice whispering, "Please, I need help. I need help."

As I repeated the words to myself over and over I started to feel calm. The tears slowed to a trickle. My breathing slowed down.

I felt a pull in that moment to talk to my mom. She knew I still struggled with food and weight loss, but I was sure she had no idea how far over the edge I had gone. I found her lying in her bed reading.

"Oh, honey, what's wrong?" she asked when she looked up and saw my tear-stained face.

I couldn't tell her I'd been puking my guts out for over a year or that I barely ate. I couldn't even imagine her disappointment. I was supposed to be the girl going after the dream, the one with so much potential, the one that had her head on straight. I think I said something about being stressed out and disappointed about the outcome of some random audition. It wasn't the whole truth, but in many ways, I wasn't lying.

"It's so hard; what you do. Sometimes I think it's too much pressure." She hugged me. Then she said, "You know, I've been reading this book that I think will help. You should read it. like this woman."

She sorted through the stack of books in the nightstand, and then pulled one out and handed it to me. "Here it is!"

"*The Gift of Change* by Marianne Williamson." I said, reading the title. "What's it about?"

"You'll see. I like how she says things. It makes life make sense."

I went back to my room and flopped down on the bed. My mother had also given me a small jar of hormone cream with instructions to put a little on my wrist. She said it would balance me out. I did as I was told. I put on a little hormone cream, and I started reading. I doubted a book was going to help. Would it feed me? Make me think I was thin, beautiful and talented?

But as my eyes scanned the pages each word made perfect sense. The book seemed to be speaking directly to me in a profound way. Based on the teachings of *A Course in Miracles*, something I had never heard of before, this book presented a way to look at change as an opportunity to receive the gift of personal transformation. Marianne Williamson delves into the thought that the only real failure in life is the failure to grow from what we go through. It was the help I had been asking for.

When I got home the next day, I told Jeffrey what I had been putting myself through. It was not an easy conversation. He was angry at me for being so cavalier about my health and my body. He was hurt that I had lied to him countless times about my problem, telling him I was fine. More than anything he was sad that I hadn't asked him for help or let him know what I was going through earlier.

In the months that followed, I learned more about how to deal with my eating disorder than any other time in my life. I did the hard work of learning to love myself enough to want to eat and to want to live. Inspired by Marianne Williamson's book, I started doing the meditations in the workbook of *A Course in Miracles*. The meditations kept me on track and kept me sane as I breathed into the words before me on the page every morning. Each meditation seemed to reverse the way I had been thinking for most of my life. I learned to forgive myself for having gone through the eating disorder and to stop blaming others for whatever part I felt they may have had in it.

What I didn't know was that moving to Chicago that fall and beginning my yoga practice would be the final piece of the puzzle. What I was to discover when I started practicing was something that would heal me "from the inside out, bones to the skin, from the fingertips to the toes."

Beautifully Broken

From the Blog: August 18, 2015

You always assume you are the only one that needs fixing. You walk into the hot room ready to battle another ninety-minute class, laying out your mat with a sigh as you anticipate what's to come. The other students that surround you seem to have more energy, more understanding of the practice, and in every way, look like perfect yogis — the ladies in cute shorts and tops with an obligatory messy-but-not-too-messy topknot in their hair, and the men in their tech tees and Fitbits at the ready. You've gotten better at trying to fit in, but if everyone knew why you showed up to class day after day, they would understand that you are different. You are broken and you are trying to get fixed.

I'm going to tell you a little secret: *Everyone* is broken and trying to get fixed. That girl in the front row with the perfect body is in pain throughout most of the class and masks it with a smile as she works to heal her injury. That guy who saunters into the studio and knows everyone by name, has depression and lives alone. The woman who always seems so freaking happy all of the time lost her daughter last year and is learning to cope with her loss. The marathoner always wearing his latest race tee, had surgery two months ago and came right to the studio after his physical therapy session. The size eight used to be a size fourteen. The extreme back bender used to have back problems. And even the most flexible yogis in the room, who might be able to pull off some impressive postures, have holes somewhere in their lives.

I honestly believe we are here on this planet, in this life, to work for something better than before. Maybe not to fill up our holes, but to find a way to see the holes, acknowledge them, and work our way through them. Yoga is one of the tools we have to work through this stuff. It's certainly not the only tool out there, but it is an awesome tool.

I often hear students proclaim that they wish they were better — better people, better yogis, in better health, and better at relationships of all kinds. This is actually a great thing. They are looking to be better and do better and this makes them one step ahead of most of the world out there.

Why do you think you are the only one out there seeking your highest Truth and your best Self? Why do you think you are the only one that struggles in the hot room and with the yoga practice itself? You are not alone. You are surrounded by different packages of the same broken pieces.

In the hot room, teachers often talk about how we share each other's energy throughout class. They encourage students to try and refrain from taking a break, being a distraction, or (horrors!) leaving the room. Why? Well, for ninety minutes we are all the perfect fit for what others in the room need, and any less than that will make the overall energy of the class take a dip. Even the newbies in the back, wondering how everyone else is doing this crazy yoga, are contributing to the energy. They make us all reflect back to that time when we were the newbies and, in turn, we send them positive vibes of support and compassion.

When I am having a rough practice, lacking balance and concentration, I consciously glom onto the stronger yogis surrounding me. I fall out of a posture and then re-enter it, thinking of the image of the person on the mat in front of me holding it with strength and grace, and suddenly I am also holding it with a new level of ease. It's a trick I will use for the rest of my life, for we are all connected in some way while we sweat it out day after day.

I also use this trick in my life outside of the hot room. When I begin to worry about something or have a situation go in the wrong direction, I picture how the positive people in my life might deal with the situation or imagine what they might say if I asked them for advice. I know that, whatever I may be lacking, the way to resolve this lack is shown to me in the faces that surround me every day. The people in our lives are there to teach us how we want to be (and how we don't). The tricky part is accepting the lessons.

I guess the message I'm trying to impart is that nobody is better off in the hot room than the next. We are all simply trying our best — in the studio and outside of it. There is no need to be intimidated or to think that you are the only one who is in some way or another "broken." In fact, over time you might find that what you once thought of as broken was actually the perfect vehicle for you to make the changes that have you becoming the person you always knew you could be.

CHAPTER FOUR

REWRITING THE SCRIPT

In February of 2006, I arrived in Arizona, cast once again as a showgirl. I hadn't been able to say no to the job when it had been offered to me a few months before. It was good for my résumé, it was at a theater where I enjoyed working, and seemed like a perfect role to dive into for a couple of months. The one negative was that Jeffrey wouldn't be able to make it out to see the show - February through May were his busiest months at school, since he was music director for the spring musical. That meant ten weeks apart. Sometimes I hated that I loved my job.

John, the stage manager for the company, was waiting for me at the curb outside baggage claim. He smiled and wrapped me in a big hug. "Welcome back! We're excited to have you on stage with us again."

"I'm looking forward to it too!" I said, my smile a little forced. I was excited but nervous about the weeks ahead.

The last time I had worked at this theater, for the holiday show in 2004, I had been a wreck - hardly eating, exercising too much, getting thinner and thinner by the day. I had felt an immense amount of pressure at this theater, because everyone cast in the shows seemed already perfect and talented. They were the sort of performers who had the luxury of a whole year of shows booked at a time, knowing when and where they would be. I had felt I had to prove, that I, too, was already perfect and talented.

My wish this time around was that I could prove to myself that I could do this without puking my guts out every chance I got or starving myself into a smaller costume. As I gazed out the car window at the mountains, the blue sky, and the warm sun - such a contrast to the gloom and doom of a Chicago winter I had left that morning - I told myself I would be okay. It would be different this time, because I was different. I had changed. I was healing.

John dropped me off at the hotel and gave me my welcome packet. After I settled into my room, I opened the thick manila envelope, which contained the rehearsal schedule, cast list, script, music, theater rules, and a map of the local area (so that out-of-towners could find the nearest grocery story or sandwich shop easily). I scanned the cast list. I had worked with almost everyone before, except for a few of the ensemble members. The familiar names were people that either knew I had an eating disorder or highly suspected it. This would not be a fresh start by any means.

"I am different though, so maybe these relationships will be different," I thought.

The door opened and a distinctive voice called, "Hey, Tor! We're rooming together for rehearsals! Cool!"

Kate, the actress who would be playing the lead, pulled a huge suitcase into the room.

"Hi!" I smiled and gave her a hug, but my stomach tied itself into elaborate knots.

The last time I had worked with Kate I couldn't wait until the curtain dropped on our final show. She had made my life a nightmare. In a chance accident on stage, I had sprained my ankle and scraped my legs. After seeing a doctor to make sure I didn't have a hairline fracture, I was told I couldn't perform for three days. Kate thought I was lying. My being sidelined ruined one of her laugh lines in the show, as my presence on stage made it work. She tried to make me feel guilty about being injured, and I had caught her more than once talking badly about me with others in the cast. I had thought she was a friend. We had worked together lots of times, and it hurt to have her words affect the way the rest of the cast saw me.

Now I had to spend two weeks in a hotel room with her. It would be the ultimate test to see if I had changed. If I could forgive Kate and see her in a new light by the end of this, I would be proud of myself. If I could be around her and not start feeling like I needed to head to the bathroom to throw up after a meal, that would be even better.

At the start of rehearsal the next day, I was apprehensive, yet happy to see old friends and work with them again. There was new choreography to learn and new songs to sing, and I was ready for the work at hand. I walked into the rehearsal hall and took a seat in one of the chairs that had been set out for our first meeting, having to stand up over and over again to offer a hug to the actor I was partnered with in my last show, the actress I had roomed with a few years earlier, and to meet and greet the actors that were new to me.

After the initial meet and greet, we gathered around the piano, plunging into music rehearsals and starting the process of making the words on the page come alive with the sounds and voices that made up the company of characters we would be playing for the next ten weeks.

When we had a lunch break, I ate lunch. I was hungry and knew I needed the fuel to keep me going. Preparing for the afternoon choreography session with a full stomach felt strange. I was so used to doing this without the heavy feeling of food grounding me, but I found moving through the rehearsal with a different kind of energy that I enjoyed, feeling centered and solid as I began to memorize the choreography to the opening number.

The ten-day rehearsal period seemed easier than most. Every morning I would wake up long before Kate and pull out my copy of *A Course in Miracles*. Sometimes I had to meditate sitting on the toilet in our bathroom with the door locked, and other days I went outside and sat on the steps by the hotel pool. I needed those meditations even more than before.

The meditation and taking care of myself and the fact that my blood sugar levels were normal (because I was eating regularly) meant that I no longer felt overly emotional or stressed out. The role I was playing was a perfect fit for me, so I wasn't striving to be something I was not, but was enjoying the role and the challenges it brought up as we moved through the rehearsal process.

The relationships with my fellow actors, on the other hand, weren't as easy. It was difficult to weed through my past feelings for these people and see how they were making me feel now that I was in the process of healing. For years I had slowly ripped myself apart in front of them, and now the colleagues closest to me had started to notice the positive changes. Some were happy for me and loved to see me happy. Others did not seem to like this new healthy version of me.

I was supposed to be the messed-up friend. Some people like that. It makes them feel better about their own lives when they can point to someone close to them and think, "At least that's not me." Some like the idea of rescuing the messed-up friend. Being in on the action of the dramatic spiral of someone's breakdown can be strangely appealing.

This time in Arizona woke me up to the fact that in order to live the life I wanted to live, I had to distance myself from some of these relationships, Kate included. These were not bad people, but I wasn't going to get better and stay better by having them in my everyday life. Being around them made me realize that some of these relationships didn't make me feel great about myself at all. I would leave a conversation, a break from rehearsal, or a night out to dinner feeling weighed down somehow - and it wasn't because I was eating.

It wasn't easy to untangle myself from these relationships, but slowly I started to make different choices each day that led to them shifting and changing. At times, it felt kind of cruel to decline the invitation to dinner or to not take the phone call in between shows, but I also knew that it was the best choice for me under the circumstances. Some of these people had been absolute fixtures in my life. They were the girls I would talk to every day about something or other, no matter where we each were currently performing across the country. They were the guys who would join me on a walk or grab a beer with me at the local bar to unwind after the show. But I found that just because we were friends working toward similar goals in our careers didn't mean that they were good for me, or that the relationships supported the positive life I was working towards.

The show playing before ours came to a close a few days before our opening night, and its cast, who had been living in the condos owned by the theater, left town for their next gig. I moved out of the hotel room I was sharing with Kate and into a condo I would be sharing with four other actresses. I had my own room, which would give me the privacy I desperately craved for my morning meditations and general well-being.

Kate didn't pay me much attention, now that we weren't roomies, but was consumed with making sure that everyone else around adored her. She had a habit of pulling people in with witty jokes and an abundance of compliments (that didn't quite seem sincere if you were paying attention). My gut told me to stay out of her way, so I didn't make myself available to spend extra time with her. We could co-exist and work well together without having to be overly involved with one another.

Once the show opened I had more time to myself. I found the local Bikram Yoga studio and went at least once a week. It was my home away from home with the familiar salty smell of sweat in the air. I would slip off my shoes and unroll my mat in a sunny spot by the front window and breathe a sigh of relief that I had been able to get there. The same postures, the same heat, and the fun of having a whole host of new teachers to learn from made it a welcome oasis through the weeks of performances. The yoga seemed to center me in a way that nothing else could.

The theater had a cast car that we could sign out and use to help us get around town. It was challenging to get the car for a full two and a half hours to ensure that I had time to get to the yoga studio and back. Knowing I wanted to take class on Tuesday mornings, I'd sign the car out in advance as soon as it was made available to us. The studio was far enough away that if I couldn't get the cast car, I couldn't go to yoga. I talked another actress into coming with me sometimes, so she would sign out the car on Friday mornings.

Having performed in Arizona time and again, I had friends among some of the local actors. One of them, Heidi, wanted to get everyone together while I was in town. She invited me to a girls' night at her house. She knew what it was like to be stuck in cast housing for weeks on end, the monotony of wiling the hours away until it was time for the next performance. Mondays are typically an actor's only day off, so she picked me up on Monday evening and took me back to her place.

A few moments after we arrived at Heidi's home on the other side of the valley, the other girls arrived. I was excited to see everyone and catch up. There were six of us altogether, and I was most excited to see Gabby, one of my closest friends at the time. We talked on the phone most days (lately the timing was closer to weekly instead of the everyday thing it had once been).

Gathered together in the family room, we drank wine and talked about our boyfriends and husbands. We chatted about how my show was going. We gossiped about the actors we had all performed with before and what they were up to now. We talked about upcoming auditions and dreamed about being cast in certain shows. It was a fun night.

As we were talking about the new theater that had recently opened in a neighboring suburb of Phoenix, I mentioned that I wasn't planning to audition for shows there anytime soon, because there were still a lot of kinks to work out. (Other actors I knew had hated their experience working there: there were a variety of technical problems, the rehearsal process hadn't been worked out, and the theater had yet to bring on the directors and choreographers needed to make it a successful venue.) I was just sharing my opinion, right or wrong. I had felt comfortable surrounded by friends I had known for years and didn't think I had to watch everything I said. But the energy in the room suddenly changed.

As soon as the words left my mouth I knew I had offended Gabby. She had recently finished a show at that theater and wanted to work there again. For her, it was work close to home. She could perform and not leave her boyfriend for weeks. I understood that. If I could work close to home and be with Jeffrey all of the time, I would. But I also wanted to have my résumé reflect good work at good theaters. I tried to brush it off and started talking about something else, hoping to shift the energy back to something fun and positive, but when I left that night I knew that Gabby was unhappy with me.

The next afternoon as I was walking the mile from the condo to the theater, enjoying the sun and the mountains in the distance, and mentally preparing for another performance, my phone went off. I looked at the name on the caller ID. It was Gabby. I took a breath and picked up the call.

"I think we need to talk," she said, flatly, but in a moment her voice rose to an all-out holler. "I can't believe you said last night. I'm furious. It's hard to get work out here. Who are you to turn work down if it's offered?"

The litany went on and on.

I listened quietly to what Gabby had to say until she was done. Then, I took a full breath and let it go.

"I didn't mean to offend you. For me, what I said was the truth: I would not work there right now. Working there would mean leaving Jeffrey and home for another ten weeks, and I can only do that so often anymore and claim that I still have a marriage that works. I understand why you want to work there. You live here. It makes sense. I love you and don't want to hurt you."

Silence on the other end.

"Are you still there?" I asked finally, wondering what was going on.

"I didn't expect that. I thought you would yell back."

"I don't want to do that to you. We have different opinions. Isn't that okay?"

"Of course. But when you said you wouldn't work there, I felt as if you were saying that actors who would weren't as talented. That we were mediocre."

"That wasn't what I was trying to say at all. Down the line, I'm sure I'll find myself begging for work there, but right now it's not the right fit."

I could almost hear her taking my thoughts into consideration.

"Are we okay?" she asked, "You're so different lately."

"Sure. Things are just changing for me right now - and it's a good thing they are. You know that."

"I know. You looked better last night. Happier."

"Thanks. I'm working on that," I replied. "It was good to see you. Talk soon?"

"Yeah, talk soon."

I actually was changing. Before I would have cried and hollered - even standing on the sidewalk with my cellphone - but instead I had calmly laid out my point of view and communicated as best I could. Even so, I was a bit sad. I had the feeling that even though we had set things straight and they seemed okay, Gabby and I were growing apart. In many ways, the distance between us had been growing over the past months, as the time between our phone conversations had grown from a few days to a week to a few weeks. This would turn out to be one of our last conversations. Our energies didn't match anymore. Before I had been on a constant rollercoaster ride of emotions, and Gabby was a friend who tried to save me from myself when I was at my worst. We had cried and laughed a lot. There was very little even ground and what I needed right now was even ground.

The rest of the run was uneventful. The cast had gotten used to the fact that I kept to myself. I would wake up earlier than the other actors I lived with, meditate, and then go for a quick three-mile run (or to yoga), shower, and have some cereal for breakfast. If we didn't have an afternoon performance, I would read or watch movies on my computer in my room, making a sandwich for lunch or taking a walk to grab something at a nearby restaurant. Sometimes I would sit outside by the pool. When it was time to go to the theater, I'd grab my dance bag and start walking, rather than waiting to squeeze into the cast car with the other actors.

The performances went well. I enjoyed the choreography and had fun with my role. I had also booked up some work for the summer, so I didn't feel pressured to find more work once this show closed. Like so much of my life during the years when my eating disorder was the worst, my need to appear perfect while at this theater had been a warped perception of the truth. I had discovered that the more I worked to be the most authentic version of myself, the more everything in my life seemed to be falling into place.

**

After three short months at home with Jeffrey, I packed up my car for the drive to that next job for two summer stock shows at a theater in downstate Illinois. The good part: once the first show opened, I would be performing that one at night and rehearsing for the next one during the day, leaving me very little free time to feel lonely or bored. The bad part: I had worked at this theater before and, as with the one in Arizona, it was difficult for me to go back.

The last time I had been there, my eating disorder had been out of control. I had been housed in a typical dorm-style room with one great amenity: a private bathroom. That had made it easy to throw up - and not be discovered - whenever I had to eat with the cast or with my family and friends who came down to see the show.

Once again, I had to face my demons.

Luckily, I met Kara on the first day. She was performing in the current show and would be in the next two shows with me. She was striking - with long honey-colored hair and dark brown eyes - talented, and, best of all, down to earth. She took the time to talk with me on breaks during rehearsals, and there seemed to be an instant kinship between us. Kara reminded me of my younger sister, as they were about the same age. She was from Iowa and had the same kind of Midwest upbringing that I did, which made it easy to relate to each other. A week into rehearsals she confided that she was in a nightmare of a roommate situation. Her roommate was twenty years her senior and bossy as well as a slob. I was staying in a two-bedroom apartment by myself, and I was finding it more isolating than any other cast-housing situation I had ever experienced. Taking a leap of faith, I told her that she could move in for the remainder of her contract if she felt it would be a better fit, and she leapt at the chance to make the switch.

It was good to have Kara around. She was normal. She ate doughnuts for breakfast. I needed her that summer. We would grab meals together between rehearsals and shows. We'd watch bad reality TV when we came home at midnight or first thing in the morning before rehearsal. There was no extra drama with Kara. I knew she would never talk badly about me or waste time on petty gossip. I could be normal around her and laugh. We both believed in the work we were doing and wanted to have fun performing.

From ten a.m. until eleven-thirty p.m., each day was crammed with scheduled rehearsals and costume fittings, and squeezing in one last dance or music rehearsal whenever time was available, before rushing to call times for matinee and evening performances.

The daily routine didn't offer much free time, but I still made it a priority to continue my morning meditations, as they helped set me up for the day. Meditating always reminded me I was good enough. In that moment I didn't have to conform to whatever tricks my mind might play on me when I felt I was falling short in rehearsals or when I started getting critical of my reflection in the rehearsal room mirrors.

There was no yoga studio in the area, so I would go for a two- or three-mile run in the morning and then work on some of my postures outside the apartment, watching my form in the reflection of the patio doors.

Jeffrey drove down to see each show and spend a little time with me, taking me out to lunch or dinner on my breaks and applauding loudly when I came out to take my final bow. It seemed luxurious to have him there twice.

The days melted into one another, and it seemed that as soon as I started rehearsals, we were already closing the second show. We packed our things the next day, and I gave Kara a hug goodbye.

As I drove towards home and Jeffrey through the miles of southern Illinois cornfields, I thought about my successful run - on and off stage. I felt certain now that I could perform without going back to the old habits of my eating disorder. The two didn't have to go hand-in-hand. The meditation and the yoga had changed me in a way nothing else could. I understood that every positive choice I made each day had begun to add up to one incredible life, filled with new friends, a husband who loved me, and a career I still adored.

MAT TO MAT CHAT

DAVID

When I first noticed David in my classes I was aware of his commitment to his practice, his determination as he approached each posture, and - his bag of ice. Here was a student who came to class five or six days a week, but he was distracted by the heat in such a way that he looked for solutions to find comfort in the hot room. He'd rub an ice cube onto his face or grasp one in his hand during Savasana. Comfort is not what a yoga asana practice is about. It is honestly the most uncomfortable thing you can pursue for a myriad of good reasons.

I didn't say anything at first. I let it continue for a couple of months, observing when he would grab for his ice and why. I waited until we'd gotten to know each other a bit. Then one day he began talking to me about the yoga practice and I saw my opening. I mentioned the bag of ice cubes.

He blushed. "I wondered how long I was going to get away with that."

"I think it's time to let it go. You have a strong practice. It's hot in there, but you can handle it. The ice isn't helping anything. See if you can leave it behind."

Next time I had David in class he had let it go. The ice had disappeared and his focus became sharper. The distraction of clinging to something cool in the heat had become part of his past, which, I came to realize in the years we practiced together, held much more.

David had started practicing Bikram yoga a couple of years before I met him while he was in Japan on business. He had even taken classes taught by Bikram Choudhury. But he had discovered yoga much earlier, in the Seventies while spending time in a halfway house for drug and alcohol addiction as a teenager.

"I loved it. It changed me. We'd get up early on Saturday mornings and meet one of my counselors. We'd do hatha yoga and then go hang out at a student union. I was fifteen and super impressionable. I was sober and clean and I was a yogi - it was something I wanted to be."

While he still struggled on and off with drug addiction, David always thought of yoga as something he liked and something that had been good for him, based on this first experience. Years later, clean and sober, a successful corporate executive, living overseas with his wife and children, he rediscovered yoga at a moment when he truly needed it.

"In Japan, I was in a tough place. I was the tenth Chief Marketing Officer for this company in ten years at this location. It was a top-ten brand, and there was an enormous amount of pressure to do well. I had come out of Latin America where I had become known as someone that was good at turning things around for a company. I was full of myself and sure it would be an easy, quick fix and then I would be out. But I got sucked into a tough assignment. And then there was an earthquake there… It was bad."

David started taking anti-depressants (a tough choice for him to make as a recovered addict). He was also diagnosed with a herniated disc in his lower back and found himself dealing with pain and discomfort like never before. Then his wife suggested he join her at a yoga class she wanted to try.

"It was a non-chemical answer to some of the issues in my life, so I thought, 'This is good.' I hadn't been in a studio in thirty years and I'm thinking I'm good at yoga. But that was when I was fifteen."

That first class, he says, was "revelatory. I thought it was over when the Standing Series ended, and I remember thinking, 'Wow that was something!'"

Thinking the class had concluded, David left the hot room as the other students lay down in Savasana (before the start of the Floor Series). With no place to sit other than the bathroom, he watched as the heat coming off his body fogged up the mirrors.

That first class "was like being in an auto accident, really loud and really jarring. It was incredibly powerful and not pleasant. Since I'd done yoga before, I thought it would be like coming back to something, whereas, this was entirely new."

After his wife finished class, they headed home, where David lay down, and woke up three hours later from one of the best naps of his life.

He was hooked. While the culture in Japan was to go out for a drink after work, David headed to the studio instead.

Towards the end of his contract, David found himself in Japan alone. He had sent his family back to the U.S. after the 2011 earthquake that shook Japan to its core, listed as one of the fourth largest earthquakes ever recorded, with almost 16,000 deaths and over 6,000 injured. He traveled back and forth, going home for three days at a time to be with his family, and toggled between a hot room in the States and a hot room in Japan.

Eventually, his assignment came to a close and he came home to stay. And he came to the studio, where he continues working hard, day after day, and - with a little push in the right direction - letting that bag of ice melt into the history of his practice.

There are certain people that make a studio special. Those people you know you will see if you go at a certain time and even if you don't know them, you know they are part of what makes a place great. David is one of those people. He's quick to strike up a conversation and is always kind and interested in what the other people have to say. He laughs often but takes his practice seriously. He makes me want to be a better teacher. I know I need to push him, but I have to do it in a way that won't frustrate him, or make him think that what he's already accomplished is nothing short of amazing.

CHAPTER FIVE

AND...CHANGE

Most of my acting career had been a juggling act. Between theater jobs I worked for a temp agency, taking assignments that lasted a couple of weeks or a couple of months with the understanding that I would have to leave work occasionally for auditions. One company began hiring me every time I arrived back in town after closing a show, whether they needed me or not, it seemed. I worked for the same team every time but in a different capacity, gaining knowledge with each role. I learned everything about their product line and the vendors they worked with, often stepping in to fill positions that wouldn't normally go to a temporary worker.

The office staff accepted me as one of the crew. Whenever I had to leave for a couple of hours for an audition or when my phone rang with a call from my agent, they responded with a flurry of excitement and encouragement. I was the office's resident actor. I was also the resident yogi, equipped with a gallon jug of water to drink throughout the day, preparing for the hot room that night.

In May of 2007, one of the copywriters resigned, and the team asked me to fill in where I could, writing product copy for the website. It was surprisingly fun. It allowed me to stretch my creative muscles in what often seemed like a very uncreative environment. And it turned out I had a knack for it.

The responsibilities of this new position expanded although I was still a temp. I found myself in frequent meetings and offering feedback and helping to make decisions and writing copy for the next email blast. In the middle of all of this I would rush off to an audition, belt out sixteen-bars of my favorite show tune, and then head back to the office. It was too much. I found myself blowing auditions, being too distracted with my office work to concentrate on the nuances of the song I was singing or the monologue I was performing. Acting was the career I was supposed to be focused on. The office gig was my side job.

One day I received another phone call from the theater in Arizona, offering me the role of Irene Molloy in a production of *Hello, Dolly!*, and I couldn't turn it down. I had played the part at another venue in 2004 and I loved it. The contract would run from the beginning of February through the middle of April 2008.

As I prepared to tell the office team I would be leaving (again) in February, I decided I didn't want this for myself. I didn't want to be better at a temporary job than I was at performing, and that seemed to be what was happening. It was either time to leave the temp job for good or to create a different situation for myself.

I asked the head of our team, Sharon, if she would consider hiring me as a consultant, allowing me work from home or wherever I was on a theater job with only occasional trips to the office. Once a show was open, my days were fairly open (and boring), and it would be nice to have writing projects to work on and to be able to make extra money on the side. I was prepared for a flat-out no, but to my surprise, she said yes and had a contract drawn up by the following day.

My return to Arizona involved a routine similar to my previous job at the theater: rehearsals, then opening the show, and then the weeks with unscheduled time each day until the performance. Now, however, I had writing projects to work on and emails to respond to from the office. I went back to the same yoga studio, enjoying that I had a home-away-from-home studio.

At the theater I enjoyed the process of putting the show together with fresh choreography and actors I had not worked with previously. As the show progressed and I became more familiar with the actors around me, I felt a sense of being older than everyone else. I wasn't the oldest member in the cast, but I had performed here over and over again, knew where everything was, who to talk to in the production staff and backstage crew about the most minute and mundane things, and I had a routine for my days that worked. The first-time cast members were enamored with being at this theater and wowed by every facet of their time there, much as I had been five years earlier.

Each time I joined another actor on a visit to a local restaurant or on a hike, a sense of nostalgia settled over me. I could recall a group I went with to this restaurant sometime before, or how I had laughed with another actor on the same exact hike three years earlier. New ensemble members would seek me out to ask if the two-hour drive out to Sedona was worth it on their Monday off or if the Grand Canyon was too far away, assuming I had done these trips in the past (which I had). It was as if I were shedding the skin of this era of my life. At the time, I wasn't sure why I felt this way. I just had a sense, a feeling, that this was the last time I would be out this way performing, and I turned out to be right.

The show closed in April, and I hadn't been home long when I received an offer to head back downstate for two shows in the summer stock season: Electra in *Gypsy* and Miss Sandra in *All Shook Up*. These roles were on my list of Must Play Before I Die or Become Too Old, so I accepted, even though the job would pull me away from home once again. Then, much to my surprise, I was offered an Equity contract for the work. Joining the actors' union is a big step forward in a performer's career, and there are two ways to join. The first is to pay dues and work fifty weeks at Equity-approved theaters, which can take years. At the time, I only had thirty-seven weeks under my belt (and thought it would take at least another three years to accrue the other thirteen). The second way is to be offered an Equity contract. An offer like this is not made often or lightly to non-union actors, so I jumped at it. Getting my Equity card was something I had dreamed about for years and worked toward with each contract and each audition.

Being an Equity actor would mean I could only work at theaters that were a part of the union and followed union rules. This would change my acting life. The theater in Arizona, for example, was non-Equity, so I would no longer be able to work there. Just as I had sensed, that chapter of my life was finished.

***

There were other changes waiting for me when I got home from Arizona.

One day Jeffrey announced, "I think we should get a dog."

His face was serious and his brown eyes wide and blinking as he looked at me with pursed lips, all signs that indicated this was something he had given some thought.

"Seriously? Don't joke with me," I said. I sat on the couch happily stunned, not wanting to move. "You know I've always wanted a dog, but that's not for me to decide. I'm gone too much. You'd be the one taking care of it most of the time."

"Babe, I'm kind of sick of being home alone. I think it would help."

Genuinely looking at him in that moment, I knew that what he was saying was true. He had never said before that he felt lonely. In fact, he often encouraged me to take jobs I turned down, telling me to go if I wanted to, and I would joke that he just wanted me out of his hair and back on the road. He was (and is) my biggest supporter.

"You're lonely?" I felt sick at the thought. I didn't want to make him feel that way.

"It's hard to come home after a long day to an empty apartment when you're gone. It would be nice to have a dog here. I think it would help."

I took his hand, gave him a kiss, and smiled. "What kind of dog?"

For a couple of weeks, we dreamed about the dog. I had suggested a pug. They were so cute and small - but not too small. That seemed like a good fit for us and our one-bedroom apartment. On the Monday of Memorial Day weekend as we were headed to the movies, we stopped into a pet shop to get an idea of what kind of dog might fit us best. We were not going to buy a dog. We just wanted to take a look.

There were two puppies we asked to hold. One was pug, just what we were looking for, but it was crazy. It was crazy when we put it down on the floor to play, and it was crazy when we picked it up, wiggling and whining in our arms. The other dog was a puggle, which I had never heard of before.

The young woman assisting us explained that it was beagle-and-pug mix. She placed the five-pound puppy in Jeffrey's arms, and the dog melted into his chest.

"She's so sweet," he said and then handed her carefully to me.

As soon as I held her, she did the same thing, melting her head with its floppy beagle ears into my chest. She looked up at me with her big brown pug eyes and began licking my chin.

When we put her on the floor, she began to run around and play, showing us her best puppy moves. Both of us laughed at her tiny fierceness.

"We have to go if we're going to make the movie, Babe," I told Jeffrey.

"Oh, yeah. Let's get going," he said, and then as if reminding himself, "We weren't going to get a dog today."

As we left the pet shop I took a last look over my shoulder at the puggle, now in her cage, looking at us with pleading eyes as we turned and walked out the door.

A few hours later as the credits rolled in the dark movie theater, our fingers and toes frozen from the air conditioning that rolled through the room, Jeffrey stood up, looked down at me still sitting in my seat and said, "Let's go get our dog."

We drove straight back to the pet shop, relieved to find our puggle puppy still there. We bought her and an assortment of puppy stuff: a crate, a collar and leash, and the dog food the shop recommended. Placing her on my lap, I marveled at her tiny paws and soft brown eyes as we made the drive home.

Despite her small size, her large personality filled our tiny apartment immediately with her curiosity and playfulness. We set her crate in the corner of our family room in between an oversized chair and coffee table and took her outside every hour, hoping she wouldn't have an accident in the house. After some searching for baby names on the Internet we decided to name her Chandi, which meant "supreme ferocious goddess" in Hindu. It was perfect.

We soon realized that the best way to potty train Chandi - and wear her out - was to walk her. She needed to be on the move. Soon we had a walk schedule, averaging three to five miles each day. Jeffrey would walk her in the morning. I would walk her in the afternoon. And then we would all walk together at night after dinner. She had a boundless amount of energy, always wanting to play. She would scramble up on my lap and stand in front of my computer to insist that I take a break from work and have some fun, which always makes me laugh. Jeffrey would take her out by the retention pond behind our apartment and race her around and around, his laugh echoing back to me inside as it bounced off the tall buildings that stood on either side of the pond.

It's strange to say, but Chandi had made us a family. Leaving for my summer stock job at the end of June was harder than normal. Jeffrey came to see each show, bringing Chandi with him, much to the delight of my other cast members. She seemed to make everyone fall in love with her instantaneously. And by the time I got home Chandi was a fully trained dog. Jeffrey had taught her to heel and to ring a row of jingle bells hanging on the door to let us know when she wanted to go out. She would also ring them when she was bored and wanted to play or if she was hungry, but at least we knew she needed something. I guess she had trained us too.

***

Another change was that Jeffrey had given up his yoga practice. He claimed he was bored with it. One night while I was in Arizona he was taking class, and when the teacher had instructed everyone in the first forward stretch to pull on their heels as much as possible (just the same as in every other class), Jeffrey simply didn't want to anymore.

He had recently finished his master's degree and planned to go on to get his Ph.D., which would take a lot of his time and energy. Also, he had become interested in Vipassana Meditation and wanted to do a ten-day sit at a meditation center in northern Illinois. He had other things he wanted to accomplish and I understood that, though it was hard for me to wrap my head around the fact that the man who had been at the studio five or six days a week wasn't going to practice anymore.

My practice shrank down to two or three classes a week. Then, as Jeffrey started to tackle his Ph.D. work, I decided that maybe it was time for me to try something new, too. I thought I would try other types of yoga. There had to be more than Bikram Yoga, right? I drifted from studio to studio, trying out Vinyasa, Iyengar, and Flow classes. I tried to be enthusiastic about them, but I didn't understand why an instructor would walk into the room, look at her students, and ask what they wanted to work on. Shoulders today? Hips? My mind would chatter with thoughts about how it would be nice to work on everything. That's what I showed up for. With each class I could feel my enthusiasm wane, and I finally abandoned yoga completely. I went back to daily running instead, registering to run two half-marathons and a slew of other shorter races during the next year as a way of keeping it interesting and setting new goals for myself.

Life was good. I was busy. My copywriting work fit nicely with auditioning for theater work. My marriage was healthy. I was healthy. I didn't even miss Bikram Yoga.

Until I did.

I started having daydreams about going back to the hot room, thinking about what that first inhale in Pranayama Breathing would feel like as the hot air filled my lungs and my shoulders contracted. It took me about a week before I got up the courage to go back. I was worried the teachers would recognize me and be disappointed that I had been gone so long. Or even worse, they wouldn't recognize me at all.

As I climbed the stairs to the studio on a September morning, I wondered what I would find. Would I love it as much as I had before? Or had I outgrown it as Jeffrey claimed he had? When I entered, Mara, one of my favorite teachers, was at the front desk.

"You're back!" she exclaimed, giving me a big hug. "I am so happy to see you!"

I couldn't wipe the goofy grin off my face. I was literally welcomed back with open arms. The wave of heat that greeted me when I opened the door to the hot room felt like a welcome-home parade. As class began, the familiar sounds of Pranayama Breathing filled the room. I listened to the collective hum as we inhaled and the whoosh of the "hah" sound as we exhaled. I couldn't help but smile at myself in the mirror with the sheer joy of being back. This was my yoga. I was home.

The eight a.m. class became part of my schedule. Most weekday mornings Jeffrey would leave for work, Chandi would curl up in her crate, and I'd email back some of the writing I had worked on the day before, grab my bag and mat, and drive to the studio. Some days I had to skip it to attend an audition or go to a print call (something my agent insisted I start doing, because print work paid more than most other jobs), but even then I would often squeeze in my practice at a studio close to the audition in downtown Chicago. Soon it was a rare week when I wasn't on my mat in the hot room for at least five sessions, taking a break on the weekends to be with Jeffrey and Chandi.

One morning when I had been back to my regular practice for a few weeks, a woman began chatting with me in the locker room after class as she combed out and tied back her thick blonde hair.

"I started about a month ago and I'm still getting the hang of it. I don't think I'll ever be able to do Half Moon like you do," she said, smashing a black baseball cap on her head and somehow looking pulled together and perfectly pretty in one simple move. "Oh, by the way, I'm Jane."

"Tori," I replied and smiled at the friendly face before me. "You will though. It just takes some time."

Little did I know that this conversation would blossom into a daily chat. Over time, some of the other women around us in the locker room joined in, contributing to the conversation. Some days I would look at the clock and gasp, realizing that we had gabbed about yoga and life for over an hour. We'd talk on and on in the locker room, in the stairwell on our way out of the studio, or even in the parking lot.

Soon our after-class chats extended to lunches, where we could amaze each other with what we looked like with real clothes and make-up and dry, styled hair. They would ask about my latest audition, and I would ask about their kids and families and careers, learning what brought each of them to the studio day after day. Over time I realized that I wasn't heading to the studio only for the yoga, but also for the people I met there.

With this new devotion to the yoga, my practice improved. I loved the thrill of seeing my body change as I continued to rise to the commitment of a regular practice, gaining flexibility and strength in new ways. I read books on yoga, talked about yoga, and was interested in all things yoga. I attended the studio's posture clinics led by master teachers who pushed me and my practice to new limits. Jane and I, wide-eyed at the intensity of it all, practiced side by side (as we still do to this day), sharing the energy and the yoga, and becoming life-long friends.

It had been a year since I had booked my last show. When I finally landed one, I was thrilled. The job - in another production of *Hello, Dolly!* - was at a union theater a few hours away, which meant I could come home on my day off. It was perfect - except that I had never gone a whole year without performing, and I was concerned I might not have the stamina for the long rehearsal period.

That seemed like a good reason to embark on a thirty-day yoga challenge, something I had always wanted to try. A thirty-day challenge is exactly that: thirty classes in thirty days. Ideally, it means yoga every day, because missing a day means taking two classes in one day to catch up. It's the marathon of yoga and no joke. Counting out the days before I would leave for the theater job, I found had more than enough time to get it done and still have a couple of weeks after the challenge to recuperate and get ready to leave.

The first five days were a breeze, business as usual. But on day seven I suddenly felt how challenging the challenge was. I lay on the couch Sunday afternoon after class, looking wearily at my aching limbs.

"Why am I doing this to myself?"

"Honestly, Babe, I have no idea," Jeffrey said, shaking his head and smiling. "But you'll make it through. You always do when you set a goal for yourself. Maybe it will get easier?"

"Here's hoping," I replied.

I was amazed at the support I received. Mara and the other teachers frequently checked in on my progress, giving me tips on what to eat and drink, and how to rise above the endless ache of sore muscles. Jane helped me keep track of the days, announcing each one when she saw me enter the studio and wrapping me in a hug.

At the halfway point, it became easier. The yoga seemed to kick in and give me what I needed. I had a surplus of energy. The endless chatter of my mind died down. I felt centered and at ease with myself in a way that I had never experienced before.

On day thirty I couldn't believe it was done. I was still in Savasana at the end of class when Jane turned her head toward me and whispered, "You did it! Congratulations!" I beamed back. I felt stronger than ever and ready for the next chapter of my acting career to start.

Then I woke up on day thirty-one. As Jeffrey grabbed his backpack, gave me a quick kiss, and headed off to an early morning choir rehearsal, I felt a bit lost. What was I going to do with the time? I grabbed my gear, got in the car, and drove to the studio. And I continued with the challenge until I had to leave town for the acting job. My thirty-day challenge lasted forty-five days.

Off to my next gig I went, content in my thinking that this would be the beginning of a long string of work ahead after such a long break away from the stage. I was ready to step into Irene Molloy's shoes and her world again, ready to sing her tunes and dance her dances.

Unfortunately, the entire experience was far from what I had dreamed. The show's director had a habit of screaming at his actors when he got frustrated during rehearsal. In cast housing, I was rooming next door to a loud, drunk, too-old-for-this-kind-of-behavior actor from the current show, which meant sleepless nights for me as he shouted through the walls. The actor playing my romantic interest was sweet, but we had zero chemistry on stage, and once the show opened every reviewer called it out. The job was one of my worst experiences as a professional actor.

I made do though. Each day in the hot room had taught me not to let anything steal my peace. So, I dealt with each situation, paid attention to my breath, woke up each morning, sat for meditation, did my yoga, and took care of myself first.

What was most interesting to me was how much I had changed since the last time I had performed. I had always put up with anything in the hopes that the theater would hire me again. I'd smile through bad choreography, wretched relationships, and crazy actors, never letting others know that anything got under my skin. Now, nothing was getting under my skin. This time I watched my fellow actors groaning about our work environment, while at the same time trying to position themselves for another role at the theater, and it boggled my mind. I knew I would fulfill the contract, and I knew I would never want to work there again. Life is too short to spend time chasing bad situations.

Each Sunday night, as soon as the curtain dropped, I would trek home, driving the three and a half hours after a two-show day, so I could wake up in the same bed with Jeffrey and see him off to school Monday morning. Then I would get to the studio for my eight o'clock yoga class, write for a couple of hours, walk Chandi, and have dinner with Jeffrey. On Tuesday morning, I'd tear myself away and drive back to the theater for another week of performing. I was beginning to realize that a life in theater was no longer my passion.

***

When the show closed, I gratefully returned home. Jeffrey was in the thick of his Ph.D. work, organizing his thoughts for his thesis. Chandi would sweetly tuck in next to my left hip and fall asleep as I worked on the latest writing project. I still went to my voice lessons and Shakespeare classes and continued to audition, to book print jobs, and to go on casting calls. And, of course, I happily went back to my regular yoga practice.

About six months later I had one of those pivotal experiences. As I was collecting my things at the end of class a woman approached me. I had seen her at the studio a couple of times over the past few weeks. She was always quick to smile and say hello, but I had yet to talk with her or learn her name. We were the only ones left in the hot room.

"Can you walk me through Standing Bow Pulling Pose?" she asked. "I don't get it and you seem to."

"Oh, I'm not a teacher."

"That doesn't matter."

So, I asked her to show me the posture. She stretched up and kicked back until her torso was parallel with the floor. It was a good start. I made some suggestions, and she made the adjustments. Her back bent, her shoulders stretched, and her standing leg stayed straight and solid.

"Thank you!" she exclaimed, coming out of the posture. "That really helped."

"It looked great!" I said, almost as excited as she was. "But have a teacher look at it when you can. I'm no expert. I've just been practicing for a while."

That night Jeffrey and I went to dinner at the sushi restaurant across the street from our apartment. Between bites of spicy tuna rolls and sips of sake I told him about my encounter. I was on such a high from seeing that woman's posture improve with a few simple instructions, I could barely contain myself.

"Babe, you need to go to teacher training."

I was stunned.

"Do you realize it's a rare moment when you talk about being on stage or auditioning anymore? It's yoga, yoga, yoga, twenty-four seven with you. Maybe it's time for a change."

Over the next weeks, I found myself thinking more and more about the possibility of teaching yoga. It was like Jeffrey had given me a virus. He was right about my performing: Before it had meant everything to me, but now the yoga was moving in to take its place. I could see that looking back on my last job. And looking back to my thirty-day challenge, I could see when the whispers of becoming a yoga teacher started. My mind would spin a bit when a teacher took the time to explain the nuance of a posture during class - and I would think about how I would explain it, maybe even make the idea more accessible to the students, so they would gain more from the posture.

Some days later on our evening walk with Chandi, I announced to Jeffrey that I wanted to go to training that fall. Saying it out loud was scary. It made it more real somehow.

"This fall?"

"The spring session starts in a week. That's too soon," I said. "Do you think we can make it work?"

"If it's what you really want to do."

"I think it's what I'm supposed to do," I said, and in my heart I knew that was truth.

Deciding to Be a Yogi

From the Blog: June 7, 2016

"If you fall out of a posture, you are human. If you get back in, you are a yogi."

I have heard this phrase countless times over the years — in my first Bikram Yoga class, during teacher training, last week, yesterday. But I only honestly connected with it two weeks ago, as it came ringing from the teacher's mouth through the microphone, hitting me over the head in a new way, with a fresh meaning and clarity I didn't even know I was seeking. For years I regarded this statement as something we tell students newer to the practice to motivate them to try again, and I found that it only works with about half my students, so I very rarely use it. Instead, "Guys, you have time. Get back into the posture," is the way I deal with it, appealing to them as the partner I am and will continue to be in their practice as they hit the hot room.

Many students are turned off by the word yogi, though I'm unsure why. This is the reason I have avoided it for years. Yogi, by definition, simply means someone who practices yoga. I have had students say they appreciate not being called a yogi during class, or at the studio, as they are there to work out and sweat a ton and don't consider the class a practice that can affect every aspect of their life... yet. I have had students from India tell me that to them the term yogi refers to the spiritual men, skin dusted in white and wearing orange robes, found throughout their childhood cities, and that they are definitely not yogis.

I understand the disconnect, but this week I'm going to offer you a new way to look at it. Yoga is the study of yourself. In fact, for many of us, a yoga class is the first time we connect every facet of our Self into one being. We are the body that houses the spirit and the mind, and when we work in asana practice, or meditation, or practice the yamas and niyamas, we are closer to realizing our worth and our beauty.

When you commit to a regular yoga practice, you may find you can let go of the goals of perfectionism (they're not what is needed anyway). You came here, to this planet, to be your Self. Not perfect, but perfectly you. Deciding you are a yogi means that you know that this whole journey you are taking within the hot room is way more than a workout — it's a work *in*.

You see, I am human and I do fall out of the postures even ten years later. And, yes, I guess I am a yogi, because even though at times I feel I have nothing left to give, and my heart is beating out of my chest, I will get back in, even if I have half a second to do so before we move on to the next posture. Why is that? Because it's good for my mind. I have told myself I won't quit even when things feel uncomfortable and tough.

So, when you fall out of a posture, or simply have a wibbly-wobbly moment, decide to breathe, steady yourself, maybe even smile, and then try again. That's what being a yogi is: to realize you are not perfect and love yourself anyway *and* love yourself enough not to get mad at yourself, or beat yourself up, but to simply take the chance to try again.

CHAPTER SIX

WALKING THROUGH THE FIRE

By the time I headed to Los Angeles at the end of September of 2011 I thought I knew what to expect. It would be nine grueling weeks crammed full of yoga: two classes a day, lectures, posture clinics, anatomy classes, and long nights watching Bollywood movies. Days would start at 8:30 a.m. and sometimes go past midnight, ending around three or four in the morning. This would not be a vacation.

I had heard plenty of stories over the past six years from the teachers at my studio. They said classes ran longer than the usual ninety minutes - but what yogi hasn't taken a class that's gone over on time a bit? Some teachers had warned me that the classes were raging hot, but I thought they were just being dramatic. I was concerned about not getting a lot of sleep with the last lecture of the day usually starting a 9:30 p.m. with the occasional movie following after that. But, then again, I would be practicing more than usual, two times a day in fact, and yoga creates energy, right?

What made my head spin most with anxiety was that I wouldn't be in control. I'd have no control over the schedule, the people, the staff, or who my roommate would be. I'd have to let go and enjoy the journey. Getting through the next nine weeks would mean having to take care of myself better than I ever had before. There would be no way to make it through without proper nutrition. Eating was a basic necessity to accomplish the goal that was in front of me. I could not slip back into old patterns that might make me feel better for a moment, but that over time would make me weak and send me home early.

It had been years since my eating disorder had consumed me, though I was aware that it was always there. But I was different. I respected my body. The yoga had taught me that. Training was going to be challenging, but I was up for the challenge. I wasn't worried about my eating disorder, and neither was Jeffrey. We both knew that what I wanted more than anything was to take the podium and teach yoga.

I knew that there was one thing I could control, and it could make teacher training easier if I took care of it ahead of time: The Dialogue. Throughout training it would be my job to memorize The Dialogue and deliver each posture's script verbatim in front of my fellow trainees and the staff in posture clinics.

When I received my copy of the Dialogue in the mail six months before training, I flipped through the thin packet of pages stapled at one corner. "Easy," I thought, "I've memorized tons of scripts in my life. This won't be much different."

Well, it was very different. Everything in The Dialogue begins with command verbs. No sentence in starts with, "Well, guys could you please grab your heels?" It's just "Grab your heels," no ifs, ands, or buts about it. And the grammatical errors throughout The Dialogue drove me crazy, making it even harder to get the words into my head. I'd mentally correct it, only to have to go back over and over again to train myself to say what was written, even though my mind labeled it as wrong.

Memorizing The Dialogue was a feat unlike anything else I had ever experienced, or ever will experience. It was like a ninety-minute play in which I never stop speaking. I devoted myself to memorizing The Dialogue from start to finish, so that the words were seared into my mind. I knew the tricks I used when memorizing lines for a play would not work here - then I could rely on having other actors respond to what I said, giving the scene a shape I could reference if the words slipped away. Instead, I treated learning The Dialogue much like I treat learning new music for my repertoire. I created a recording of The Dialogue and played it in a constant loop when I was in my car or cleaning the house. I would chant along with it as I went from place to place throughout the day. Hours of my life were spent in pursuit of memorizing the words for each posture, so that I didn't have to worry about them once I arrived in Los Angeles.

The week before I left for training I was so well memorized that Mara, who was now managing the studio, allowed me to lead a mock class. She knew how hard I had worked and had let me take the podium a few times during her class to lead one or two postures at a time to get the hang of it. A mock class is a rehearsal to see how things go on the podium before a new teacher starts with the general public. Mara told me that if I did it now, I wouldn't have to do it when I came back from training. Instead I could be on the schedule and ready to teach.

The thought of doing the mock class early was exciting and daunting. It would be great to have it done and over with, but I had yet to go to training. Finally, I told Mara I'd try. The worst that could happen was that it wouldn't go well and I'd have to do it again when I returned home.

The day before the mock class I asked to have the hot room to myself on the off hours at the studio. I rehearsed for the rehearsal, teaching an empty class. It took a little under two hours, and it helped me realize where I was losing time in the words or what postures needed a little extra attention before I said them to live people the following morning.

Mara, Jane, and all of my friends from the eight a.m. class attended to support my first attempt at teaching. Taking the podium, my heart pounded as I looked at the row of the eight bodies in front of me. What was I doing up here?

We began, as every class begins, with Pranayama Breathing. The words tumbled out of my mouth, and the students moved accordingly. I was relieved as each posture's directions came out and through me and shocked at the amount of sweat that dripped down my body as I taught. My throat felt dry and scratchy for last the four postures, my vocal chords shocked at the amount talking that I was asking them to endure. When I finished with a resounding clap that signaled the end of Final Breathing, I was relieved I had made it through. The students went into their Final Savasana, and I made my way out of the room, waiting to hear what they thought.

A few minutes later, all eight came out at once and surrounded me with their smiles and encouragement. It had been fun to lead them through, and Mara deemed the class a success. I wouldn't have to do another mock class when I returned home. I knew I was going to be able to do this every day. I just had to make it through one obstacle - I had to survive training.

Packing to leave felt much like every other time I had gone off to perform. Every show contract that I signed lasted for eight to ten weeks. I had done this before, over and over again. I knew that in week five I would be homesick and missing Jeffrey badly. I knew that in week eight I'd be more than ready to come home, literally itching to board the plane.

As Jeffrey prepared a big meal the night before my flight he poured me a glass of wine. It would be my last one until I returned home, as any alcohol was prohibited at training. I sat on the couch, with Chandi tucked in beside me and Jeffrey prattling in the kitchen, and tried to breathe in the feeling of home. The smells of the cooking dinner made my stomach grumble.

The next morning, Jeffrey pulled the car up to the curb at O'Hare where he could drop me off, and we wrestled my two monstrous suitcases to the pavement. A sob stuck in my throat as I leaned into him to say goodbye. As always, I was torn between the pain of leaving him behind and the excitement for what lay ahead.

When I arrived in Los Angeles the sun was shining and a tang of excitement hung in the air. As I hauled my luggage out of the local tram and into the hotel lobby, I was looking forward to checking in, meeting my roommate, and setting up shop. Instead, I had to wait two hours for the room to be ready, only to find out there were three people assigned to a double room. It took some back and forth with staff and more time to figure this out.

A fellow trainee, hearing of the confusion, told me a nightmare story. She claimed that sometimes three people were assigned to one room, forcing them to deal with sleeping on a cot for nine weeks. I couldn't imagine that. These rooms were tiny. Two people sharing the space was going to be tight. In the end I would learn there were tons of teacher training stories like this that are either false or exaggerated versions of the truth.

When everything was settled, I finally met my roommate. Linda was from Sweden, and she had gorgeous long blonde hair and wide blue eyes, She was quick to laugh and had an ease about her that made me relax within the first few moments of meeting her. She had spent her twenties as a horse trainer and traveled to races throughout Europe. We shared that similar gypsy background of constant travel, and we had both been positively changed by our yoga practice. She had been working at the front desk of a studio in Sweden and was eager to get started with the process of becoming an instructor. We simply couldn't wait to teach.

The next morning, we had our first lecture and meet-and-greet with Bikram, Rajashree (his wife), and the staff. Linda and I made our way to the conference room that would function as our main lecture hall for the duration of training, joining the masses of people streaming out of the elevators and stairwells towards the big double doors at the end of the hall. The chatter of the people surrounding me as I anxiously entered the room was almost deafening. Several staff members with hand-held microphones instructed everyone to come in and get seated quickly. The rows and rows of chairs were tightly packed, and there was very little room to store our water bottles, book bags, and notebooks in such a compact space. At the front of the room was a small stage with a huge plush chair covered in an oversized bright orange beach towel.

As soon as everyone was seated and the room quieted down, the staff members introduced themselves. They told us where they were from, how long they had been practicing, and when they had attended training. Each person that spoke offered advice to us about how to survive the nine weeks ahead. We quietly listened, taking in what they had to say.

We were told that vegetarians would probably need to eat meat during the weeks of training. (Linda and I, both vegetarians, looked at each other with raised eyebrows.) We were told that we would have to be constantly hydrated and that once we finished one class, we must already be preparing for the next one. We would need to keep our electrolytes in check and be careful not to become depleted in any way. We were in for the ultimate yoga challenge: eleven classes a week for nine straight weeks.

Next, Rajashree took the stage. She glowed with maternal warmth and reassured us with her sweet and smooth speaking voice. She said the road would be difficult, but worth it in the end. Last to arrive, practically bounding from the back of the room, came Bikram. He exuded a natural energy and charisma as he looked out at the mass of people in front of him. He smiled and laughed as he told us that throughout the yoga classes ahead we might want to place our mats as close to the podium as possible - or as far away as we could - depending on how we were feeling. "You will feel different every day, every time," he exclaimed strutting from side to side across the stage with a knowing smile on his face.

Our first class took place that night. I filled my water bottle with as much ice as it could handle and, once again, took the elevator to the second floor. It was packed with fellow trainees, all of us clutching our yoga mats and water bottles with nervous anticipation.

One of the hotel ballrooms had been set up to function as the hot room. We had to file in a few at a time through a small entryway made of plastic sheeting. The ballroom was impressive, big enough for four hundred yogis lined up mat to mat. Mirrors spanned every side of the room, and fluorescent lights glowed from the top three feet of the walls, making the huge chandeliers that hung from the ceiling look cheap and exposed in their bath of bright light. Large plastic tubing snaked its way around the room, humming dully in the background as it released hot air into the cavernous space. Huge, industrial fans at the back of the room forced the heat and humidity to charge towards the middle of the space.

At the front of the room stood the podium, but it was like none other I had ever encountered before. It looked at least twenty-five feet high, making me crane my neck upwards to see the top, where, once again, an oversized cushioned chair draped with orange towels had been placed. Mirrors on each side of the podium reflected back to the people in front of it every corner of the room.

I confidently placed my mat in the second row with the podium looming in front of me. I was going to rock this class - I was sure of it. I had been waiting for this moment for months. And after five days of no practice (to allow my body a break before I put it through the training's regimen of two classes a day) I couldn't wait to bend and stretch in the heat. *Let's do this,* I thought.

As more and more of the trainees filtered in and chose a spot for their first class, the room filled with the raucous noise of nervous chatter, bouncing off the mirrored surfaces. Some people quietly sat on their mats, hugging their knees to their chests and observing the crowd around them. Others aggressively stretched out their limbs or carefully lined up their bottles of fluids at the side of their mats - prepared with water, coconut water, and electrolyte pack, they looked like yogi bartenders. Still others stood in groups and talked, and several languages filled my ears with the complex twists and turns of vowels and consonants.

The tension and off-the-wall energy created by so many people was something that could be cut with a knife. So was the humidity. And the heat. It was hot. Hotter than ever before. (I had heard that the temperatures soar at training to help future teachers understand what a first-time student feels like in class - and to make sure we never forget it.)

I noticed Linda coming into the room with her friends from Sweden. As she placed her mat towards the back of the room, I caught her eye and waved. She smiled back and threw a double thumbs-up my way.

Soon after, a noticeable silence descended upon the room, starting at the back and working its way forward. Glancing over my shoulder, I could see that Bikram, dressed in high-cut black trunks with his hair tied in a knot at the top of his head, was making his entrance. Everyone moved to stand on top of their mats as he made his way through the crowd. We all watched in silence as he climbed to the top of his podium. Standing in front of the big, plush chair, he looked out at us, put the headset microphone close to his mouth, and barked, "Check, check." His words echoed off every mirror in the room. Then he shouted, "Let's rock and roll!"

Suddenly I was in the midst of one of the hardest classes I had ever taken - or will ever take - in my lifetime. I was tickled by the sound of four hundred people practicing Pranayama Breathing together; all the inhales and exhales filled my ears with what sounded like a swarm of bees. But soon, my delight turned to distress. Bikram kept talking as we held Half Moon Pose for a seeming eternity (certainly longer than what the teachers at my home studio would attempt with the general public), his words looping through the Dialogue and back again. By Awkward Pose, only the second set of postures in the series, I was wiped out and had to take seat, knowing that we were only at the very beginning of this class. Every moment was physically and mentally draining. My mind searched for a way out, and I continued to tell it to stop all that chattering and try and enjoy the class.

At "party time," I grabbed my stainless-steel water bottle, finding it hot to the touch. The ice water I had prepared before class had been transformed to the temperature of a fresh cup of tea. The taste of warm water offered little relief or comfort as I glanced around at the trainees that were somehow flourishing. Then I caught the eyes of some around me who were also dying a small death in this too hot, too long yoga class.

How quickly I went from feeling like a yoga rock star to feeling like someone who had never experienced a yoga class before in my life! If I had thought about all the classes that were ahead for me before I would graduate from training, I would have quit right there and gone home. So, I decided to just make it through this one class, even if I had to take breaks, even if that humbled me beyond words to do so.

Somehow, someway I made it through, and the class finally came to an end. As I lay in Savasana I looked over at the girl next to me, her limbs haphazardly placed with little care about the correct form of the posture. "We survived," she whispered and we both smiled.

The lights were turned off, my heartbeat came back to normal, and I could hear the hum of the heat and humidifier wind down. Bikram crooned out a song for us, which I would find out later was from an album he had recorded (he was considered a popular singer in India). It seemed an odd way to finish class, but at that point I realized this was only the beginning: I had hours and hours ahead of me to log in this room. I had no hope of it becoming easier. I was only hoping I would become better.

We were told on that first day that our posture clinic time in the beginning weeks of training would consist solely of the Dialogue for Half Moon Pose. Every single trainee would have to get up and teach Half Moon Pose to three other trainees - in front of Bikram, the staff, and all of our peers.

While I had spent the greater part of my life being a spectacle for others and was used to speaking in front of people, I found this process completely nerve racking. This exercise seemed to be an audition of sorts, and auditioning was part of my everyday life instead of the odd moment that it is for most. But the difference between this exercise and an audition was Bikram Choudhury.

When I would attend an audition, the people watching rarely spoke except for a cheery hello and a thank-you at the end. I never knew how they felt about my performance until I received the phone call that requested a callback or offered me the job. Bikram, on the other hand, would say anything that came to his mind. And I mean anything. Trainees would either receive approval for having learned the words correctly, maybe with some instruction on tone of voice or pace of the words, or complete disapproval for not getting the words memorized, resulting in a highly embarrassing moment in front of our peers.

We started this exercise on the third day of training, seated once again on the uncomfortable straight-backed hotel banquet seats in the lecture hall. There was a surge of people that needed to get their delivery of Half Moon Pose Dialogue done right away. They raced to the seats that were considered the queue for the exercise, some pushing others out of the way. It looked like Black Friday at Walmart when the doors open at midnight. I didn't have the energy for that kind of madness. So, I waited. I observed. I realized there was no rush, because there were four hundred of us, and it was going to take a while - days and days actually - to get through everyone.

On day three, I decided this was the day to take my turn at the Half Moon Dialogue. I had zero make-up on, my hair was a mess, and I was wearing slouchy cover-up pants and a tank top - the exact opposite of what I had looked like at every audition for the past eleven years. Gone was any sense of glamour. I would do this as the rawest version of myself, no longer needing the approval of anyone when it came to looks or knowledge. I still had poise and confidence and that would have to be enough.

My heart started racing as I got closer and closer to the stage. Then, finally, it was my turn. I barely remember grabbing the microphone from the stand and bringing it up to my lips. I watched the three students execute Half Moon Pose in response to the words tumbling out of my mouth. I don't think I've ever been that nervous. Bikram stopped me halfway through, waving his arm in the air.

"That was good!" he exclaimed, "Would you like to teach class tonight? I want to have dinner with my daughter."

I knew he was joking, but I fired back, "Don't tempt me. I'd love to teach tonight."

He laughed, clapping his hands at my nerve.

"How long have you been practicing?" he asked.

"Six years," I replied. Six years, I thought, from that very first class to this moment.

"What took you so long?"

MAT TO MAT CHAT

AMY

Amy was suffering from anxiety and depression when she began her yoga practice, as she was grabbing for anything that might help. Her first attempt at yoga was at a studio close to the high school where she works as an English teacher - a Vinyasa class led by the mother of one of her students.

"It was as simple flow class," Amy recalls. "I felt better after class, but I was trying to make some major changes in my life."

She had already gone through a string of changes very quickly - she had gotten pregnant, then married, bought a house, and found a new job - and a few years into it all, she was feeling overwhelmed by these landmark life events that had happened in such quick succession.

"It was too much change without processing - and postpartum depression. I crashed. I was developing weird fears and phobias. I was scared of the weather. If there was a possibility of a storm, you couldn't get me to leave the house. I'd call off work. I was afraid of everything."

Amy knew she had to do something. She saw her doctor. She took prescribed medication. She tried to be happy, to look and feel healthy, but she ended up not feeling comfortable in her own skin.

One day, feeling overwhelmed by panic, she lay down on the floor in Savasana.

"My husband came in and thought I had killed myself," she recalls. "I admit, I have had my share of suicidal fantasies, but I had a young child. I had too much to live for and I didn't want to go that route."

Some of the people at her yoga studio were talking about a Bikram Yoga studio that had opened a few towns away. She was intrigued when she heard that "it's too hot, too demanding, and too intense. It sounded like everything I was looking for."

Amy recalls her first experience as shocking. The studio's hot room made her feel a bit claustrophobic - it had no windows, an extremely tall podium, and a heated floor. She describes the happiness of getting to the first Savasana and lying down on the floor only to feel "like you were being cooked."

However, once she started practicing Bikram Yoga, Amy was hooked. The changes showed, and people noticed that she looked happier and healthier.

When she credited the yoga, she says, "They would look at me strangely. I went through a phase for a while where I thought yoga can and will fix everything. That has changed over the years. I don't say too much anymore. When I hear people complain, I've learned to just let them be."

About two years into her regular practice Amy experienced another upheaval in her life. She decided to file for divorce. She and her husband had tried to work out their issues and had been to therapy, but she realized that she was changing - and that she could only change herself.

"It has to do with self-worth, what you want in life and what you think you deserve. I guess I think I deserved a loveless marriage," she explains. "I needed to work on myself. You can't change other people. When I started to feel better about myself, I realized I couldn't wait for someone to catch up to me. I felt like I had done everything I could do and that I was the best person I could be in that moment. I had honestly tried, but it was time to call it quits. It was hard and it was heart-breaking."

Amy's divorce coincided with a diagnosis of thyroid cancer, making it even more painful and giving her even greater stress. Her thyroid and part of her parathyroid were removed. She endured radiation treatments, but luckily, did not have to go through chemotherapy. She kept up her yoga practice, and fellow students at the studio rallied around her to offer support. She has been cancer-free for over five years.

"I have no thyroid," she explains, but she has retained her sense of humor. "Whenever we are in the middle of Separate Leg Head to Knee Pose and the teacher discusses the benefits this posture has for the thyroid, I always think, 'If I still had a thyroid gland, I would squeeze the crap out of it!'"

When I met Amy (after all these major life events), I could see she had flexibility, but she lacked strength in some postures, and I urged her to work in new ways to increase that strength rather than relying on the flexibility. Sometimes her hips dipped down too low in Triangle Pose, causing a misalignment in the posture and discomfort in her hips and knees. She could hit a split in Standing Bow Pulling Pose, but she struggled with the intricacies of Standing Head to Knee Pose, as it requires a good amount of core strength that has yet to be developed.

Little by little it is all coming together. She has gained strength in the few years I have known her, and her practice has a quiet determination to it that would make even the most experienced yogi envious. When her regular studio changed hands and began offering a different type of yoga, Amy took on an even longer drive to the nearest Bikram Yoga studio.

"This yoga is my medicine," she told me. "I won't mess with that."

Students like Amy positively affect the atmosphere of the studio. They teach from their own mats. Amy demonstrates to everyone around her what grace, stillness, and integrity - in and out of the postures - looks like.

"I was such a perfectionist for the longest time. Yoga helped me let that go. And it gave me friends. It's not easy to let people in.

I needed to work on my relationships and on being a little bit more vulnerable. That has been huge."

For Amy, yoga helped fix what needed to be fixed and heal what needed to be healed. Then she realized she was ready for another change.

"I was lying in Savasana at the end of class and I said to myself, 'I'm ready for love again. I'm ready to let my past go.' And it wasn't soon after that thought that I met someone."

Amy found love again because she had *already* found love - for herself.

CHAPTER SEVEN

YOGI FOUND

I had no reply to Bikram's question at the time, but now I think I know the answer. It took me those six years to get my head on straight. It took me eleven years as an actress to go from sane and structured to crazy and scattered, and then to find my way home again to somewhat sane. It took years of doubting myself and tearing myself apart to finally find the pieces to put everything back together. I spent a lifetime wanting what others had, only to realize that maybe it wasn't what I wanted after all. It took four years in the hot room day after day, ninety minutes after ninety minutes to look in that damn mirror and smile at what I saw instead of thinking, "Too fat, too weak, too talentless, too big, too tall, not enough, not enough, not enough." Any time before that moment in the fall of 2011, standing at Teacher Training reciting Half Moon Pose, I would not have been in the right place. But in that moment, I was where and when I was supposed to be.

That's not to say training was easy. Weeks two and three were the worst for me. I realized I wasn't eating enough to keep up with what was required of me physically, making me feel nauseous and fatigued most of the time. Protein shakes, fish, and eggs were things I not only craved but also needed to keep going. While in the past I had loved to feel empty, in training the empty feeling in my stomach made me uneasy. I needed food.

I would wake up early, pour my protein powder in a shaker cup with almond milk, and go out to the hallway to mix it up, so as not to disturb Linda while she slept. I would chug the thick drink down, gagging at the taste most mornings, and then start getting ready for class. After class, I would shower and then make myself a sandwich of soy meat and sourdough bread with a side of tortilla chips and salsa. At night, after the second class of the day, I would eat whatever was available on the hotel buffet, paying an exorbitant amount for overcooked fish and salad. I didn't really care, because I was too tired to make anything for myself or to go looking for something at the nearby restaurants. Eating had little to do with enjoyment and everything to do with replacing what I lost - sodium, potassium, magnesium, calcium, and protein - in the heat.

As I stumbled out of the hot room after each session I was surprised and relieved that I had survived, taking a seat on the carpet of the second-floor lobby to collect myself before heading to the elevator. At times, I would stare up at those huge ballroom chandeliers while I lay in Savasana and pray that they would come crashing down, blissfully ending my torture in a sparkle of crystal that would be a satisfying grand exit. I had heard it said that yogis who actually died on their yoga mats went straight to heaven. Sounded good to me if heaven included cool breezes and ice-cold water. But, as much as I willed them to fall, those chandeliers never responded.

In week three I found myself in the middle of what can only be called a yoga breakdown. In the Tuesday morning class, with the amazing eighty-four-year-old Emmy Cleaves leading us through each posture, I began to feel dizzy and nauseous during the Floor Series. All the loud prints of the yoga outfits around me started to blur together in my vision, making me feel even sicker. It felt like I was on a Tilt-a-Whirl carnival ride, and I could not get off or slow it down. I had to leave the room.

I had never left the hot room before. Plenty of fellow trainees had left the room during class at this point, but for me it was a matter of pride. I was stronger than that. But I wasn't. I needed to get out of there.

Somehow pulling together the final reserves of my energy, I began crawling through the mats towards the back of the hot room. Eventually, I managed to get to my feet so that I could walk to the back doors and through the makeshift plastic hallway that led to the second-floor lobby. As soon as the cooler air hit me I collapsed onto the floor and began to sob.

I cried for so many reasons. I cried because I had left the room. I cried because I wasn't perfect enough or strong enough to stay in the room. I cried because I had enough compassion for myself to know that I had to take care of myself, that I could no longer be so cruel to my body and to my whole self in the way I had in the past. I cried because I had chosen that compassion for myself over the approval of everyone else that remained in the hot room, including the staff, the senior teacher on the podium, and my Posture Clinic group members that I spent hours with each day and practiced next to each class.

The resident nurse found me in the hallway, sitting with my knees pulled up to my chest. She helped me stand and let me lean into her as she brought me to the lobby. As I wiped my tears away and slowed my breathing down she handed me a small cup of soda. My whole body responded to the sugar and fizz of it as it slipped down my throat in two large gulps. It was like fresh water must feel to a wilting, half-dead plant. My blood sugar rose almost instantly, and I felt my head began to clear as a feeling of calm came over me.

"I've never left the room before," I whispered, admitting my defeat.

"And now you have. No alarm bells went off, did they? It's not that big of a deal," she replied, smiling.

In a few short minutes I was feeling much better, and I decided to go back into class just in time for the final breathing exercise. I walked back to my mat, smiled a reassuring smile at my surrounding group members, and kneeled down, puffing out the air in quick successive breaths as instructed. Then I lay down for a long Savasana. Afterwards, as I gathered my things, I felt lighter. Whatever this experience was it felt as if I had dropped weight -

pounds of emotional garbage - I had been hanging onto. This moment, which in the past I would have viewed as a weak one, was my strongest.

The time at training changed after that. I no longer fought the routine of two long arduous yoga classes a day. The room didn't feel as hot, and the postures didn't seem as if they were being held too long. I could feel my body rise above the challenge that each class presented. I learned to focus on the breath and the moment at hand, instead of seeing each posture ahead of me dragged out from here to eternity. I had a sense of rising above the fire. I could feel that it was hot, but it didn't bother me as it had in the first few weeks. I was beginning to access what my body was capable of, while maintaining a sense of peace and acceptance of the task at the moment. My mind no longer searched for a way out, but instead dealt with what was, and it worked with my body to complete each challenge.

I became used to the fact that the final lectures of the day started a nine p.m., when I would rather be heading to bed, and found myself looking forward to them. They focused on anatomy and the philosophy of yoga and were, for the most part, entertaining and interesting. Posture Clinics, in which we performed The Dialogue for each posture and honed our teaching skills, were easy and fun because of my prep work in the months leading up to training. I started to bond with my group members, learning about their lives away from training and what had brought them to want to teach. These people were from every part of the globe - Australia,

Japan, Germany, France, Croatia, California, St. Louis, and New Orleans. We laughed about the crazy classes we were taking, sang songs to cheer each other on, and became each other's temporary family.

Most trainees had paired off with a partner or a small group of people, using every spare moment to practice The Dialogue in preparation for the next Posture Clinic. I didn't need to participate in that way and felt left behind at times. Linda was constantly going off, her Dialogue book in hand, to meet one of her friends from back home to practice the words on the beach or at the hotel pool. I would arrive at Posture Clinic to find my group members had met for class early to practice the postures that would be covered that day, but had not thought to include me as they knew I already had it down solid. Despite my advantage of having already memorized The Dialogue, it was a bit lonely at times.

The time at training felt more like six months and not a mere nine weeks. It is affectionately called the "yoga bubble" for a reason. Everyone's time and energy was devoted to thinking about yoga and attending yoga classes. I went to sleep at the end of each long day chanting the worlds of The Dialogue and would often wake up in the middle of the night with the same words running through my head. I was out of the loop of everyday life and had no idea what was going on at home, or in the world for that matter.

At times, I was pulled out of the yoga bubble to work. I would get up early and lug my laptop and phone into the front hallway for a conference call before the morning class. Or I would scramble to pull together a writing project on my half-hour lunch break, sending it off and then rushing downstairs to attend the next Posture Clinic. Work was a welcome distraction, as it gave my mind a break from The Dialogue, or anatomy, or the crazy mandatory Bollywood movie that kept us up until three in the morning.

Jeffrey, Jane, and my parents were my lifelines to the world back home. Jeffrey and I would chat at least once a day, and he would tell me about school, how Chandi was coping without me, and the fall choir concert that I had missed. Jane sent me a text every couple of days to cheer me on and ask how it was going, making me realize what an amazing friend I had found in her. My parents seemed concerned when I told them how hot each class was, but they were glad to hear things were going well and that I seemed, for the most part, happy.

As expected, week five away from home was the worst. It was the halfway point, and there was an influx of family members coming to visit their future yoga teachers. I was introduced to husbands, wives, parents, and children that were visiting for the weekend. I shook their hands, smiling, but with a pang of regret that I hadn't tried to get Jeffrey to come to L.A. for his own visit.

I complained to him during our nightly phone call and, with a surge of hope, asked him to find a way to come visit.

"Why?" he asked. "So, I can watch you sleep? You know you won't want me there once I'm in your space for a couple of hours. I miss you too, but we can make it through the nine weeks. Get through this. It's the last time we have to be apart for this long."

He was right. We both knew from past experience that having Jeffrey there would be distracting, stressful, and tiring for me. I would try to balance what was expected of me for training with wanting to entertain him after he'd made such a long trip out to see me.

And he was right that we could make it through. By the end of training I more than ached to head home: to see Jeffrey and cuddle with Chandi and have a glass of wine, to wake up in the morning and head to the studio and unroll my mat on the all-too-familiar floor with Jane practicing next to me. I wanted home more than I had when completing any of my theater contracts. I was ready to flip the page to the next chapter of my life. I was ready to teach. I had become life-long friends in Linda, and with the members of my Posture Clinic group I had laughed and cried and gone on a journey that taught me lessons I will never forget, but around week eight, as expected, I was ready to come home.

And even though the last two weeks seemed to painfully stretch time, graduation day finally arrived. The last class had come and gone on Friday night and we were done. Saturday morning seemed odd and decadently lazy without the need to wake up for the first class of the day. That afternoon I took pleasure in dressing up for the occasion, slipping on a classic black cocktail dress, curling my hair and applying make-up for the first time in weeks.

Entering the ballroom, I was amazed at the transformation. Our hot room had been deep cleaned and returned to its formal opulence to host our final ceremony. Gone were the mirrors, fluorescent lights, and towering podium. Instead the space was filled with rows and rows of chairs and a large, elevated stage. I found my group members and took a seat in our designated area. Out-of-town guests and visiting teachers filled in the center of the room. There had to be at least eight hundred people in the space.

Bikram and Rajashree each gave a speech, and some of the most accomplished yogis from our graduating class demonstrated the twenty-six postures to music. Then one by one the 398 graduates were called to the stage to receive our certificates and have our pictures taken with Bikram. Afterwards, we celebrated with food and music. It was our last time to visit with each other and say our goodbyes, for the next day we would scatter to every corner of the world and begin teaching class.

That night I called Jeffrey from the hotel room. When I heard his voice, I burst into tears. We had talked that morning and everything had been fine. I would be flying home in the morning, and we would finally be together again. Surprised by the emotion in my voice, he asked what was going on. I had to assure him that these were good tears.

I felt such gratitude for this experience. For the first time in my life I accomplished something without leaning on someone else for help. No one could have done this for me. My yoga practice and this time at teacher training were a gift I had given to myself. In the span of these nine weeks I had been able to figure out what thoughts and habits were serving me well and was forced to let go of everything else that wasn't. I had been pushed to become the best version of myself and to leave the insecurities behind. What I found is nothing that can ever be taken away from me. I found the person I always wanted to be.

What I Wish You Knew — Things You Never Realized about Your Yoga Teacher

From the Blog: October 15, 2013

They are not perfect. Your instructors are people just like everyone else, with their own insecurities, flaws, and faults. They are students of the yoga in the exact same fashion that you are, but they became so passionate about the practice they absolutely had to share it. Yoga teachers work incredibly hard to be the leaders you need us to be, but try as we might, we still get stressed out, depressed, and angry at times. Be assured that no matter what is going on in our own lives we decide to leave it behind to lift yours up during each class, hoping to inspire you to new heights not only physically, but emotionally as well.

If your teacher sits out a posture while practicing it's because she seriously needs to. Before I became a teacher, I was always confused when I would see the instructor who tried to get me not to sit down or take a break, sit out a posture in a class I was taking with them a few days later. What was that about? What I didn't realize is how depleted an instructor can get from teaching class. That instructor taking a break may have already taught two classes that day and may honestly need that time to get her breath and heart rate under control. Good teachers try their hardest never to sit out a posture, as we are striving to lead by example, but sometimes it's best for all of us to just take a seat.

Trust them. If you don't think your teachers have ever cheated during a posture, drunk way too much water, toweled themselves off every opportunity they had, or eaten the wrong thing before or after class, then you are gravely mistaken. It is only because we have had the experience of seeing how cheating during a posture only delayed its healing results, how too much water in the belly can make you feel ill, how the hand towel is more of an enemy than a friend (making the body work that much harder to create sweat) and regretting that glass of wine from the night before, that we try and educate you on how to prepare your body for and during the practice. Yoga will never be easy, but you can make it easier on yourself by trusting what the teachers say. They've been there, they want you to succeed, they want you to grow and heal.

They are not picking on you. If teachers call out a correction to you during class it is not because they have chosen to make your life hard. It's because they can see the potential in your practice. The instructors know that correcting the form of the posture puts the student on the road to creating further balance and healing in the body. We are cheering you on with each correction. Watching you adjust the posture to go past what you believe is possible for you, is one of the reasons we love what we do.

You're putting your teacher in an awkward position (no, not the posture) when you talk or gossip about another student's practice. I know that not everyone in the room during class is going to adhere to yoga etiquette or even be nice and considerate to those around them. That is not for you to worry about. This is *your* practice. When you come up to the front desk to complain or gossip about another yogi, it makes your yoga teacher uncomfortable. The person in question may have issues you are not aware of, and it is the teacher's belief that, as that student continues to practice, these issues will drop away. If I can notice that your elbow is in the wrong place in Triangle Pose, I am also aware of everything else going on in that room and will try and get that student back on track as best as I can. Remember everyone is trying his or her best in any given moment and everyone has to start somewhere.

Your yoga teacher thinks about you long after you've left the studio. That issue you discussed with your yoga teacher or posture question you had was not left behind as the teacher drives towards home. That evening your teacher opened every book, explored every chat room and available resource she has either to find you the right answer or to understand what you are dealing with, so she could better assist you. Teachers want you to have the best experience with the yoga, because they know what a powerful healing tool it can be.

No matter what your opinion is of any given teacher she (or he) is trying her best. Maybe you have an instructor you avoid like the plague. Have you taken her class lately? Usually the reason you didn't like an instructor at first will have completely vanished if you give her another try. As the yoga has changed you, it may also have altered your perspective towards that person taking you through the class. This is a job that comes from the heart and requires passion and oodles of energy. Your yoga teacher is there, so that you can become the light.

CHAPTER EIGHT

WHEN ONE TEACHES, TWO LEARN

My first morning at home, I woke up roaring with yoga energy. I had anticipated that I would want to take a break after the intense nine weeks of training, but crazy as it sounds, my body needed more yoga. I packed up my stuff and jumped into my car. It wouldn't start. Jeffrey must have let it sit during my time away. So, I rushed to the train station on the next block, doing an awkward speed walk with my mat gripped tightly in both hands and my water bottle clanking with each step. I hopped onto the train at 9:32 and off again at 9:45, and then hustled uphill three blocks to the studio in time for class.

Walking through the doors of my home studio was thrilling. The sight of the ugly lavender, beige, green, black, and brown art deco carpeting that lined the stairway, the feel of the muggy heat even in the lobby, and the faint smell of salty sweat and forced heat hit every sense of my body. I nodded at the pictures of Paramhansa Yogananda and Bikram as I passed them.

Mara wrapped me in a welcome-home embrace. "Back for class already?"

"I couldn't help it. I'm excited to be home!"

"I'm looking forward to your class tomorrow," she said. "It's going to be great!"

Taking class that day, I was struck by how different it was from those from the past nine weeks at training. I had so much space around me. I had gotten used to being packed into the hot room mat to mat, having to step on the mat next to me to do Separate Leg Stretching and Triangle Pose. When we hit the floor series, no one's feet were in my face, and I could stretch my arms out without touching my neighbor for Full Locust. The heat was a comfortable 105 degrees with forty-percent humidity instead of the raging wall of heat at training, and it almost felt cool by comparison. The postures felt light in my body, my breathing felt effortless. Everything seemed to have an ease about it, because I had grown stronger both physically and mentally since I had last practiced in this space. It was good to be back home.

The following day, I arrived at the studio early to get ready for class. Mara was there to help me with my first check-in for the students and to show me how to regulate the heat and use the microphone. She also gave me my own key to the studio. As soon as we unlocked the doors I could hear the shuffle and stomp of feet as students climbed the stairs.

It was an incredible homecoming. Every student who checked in was someone I had sweated and stretched next to for years, and they showed up that morning to support my first time taking the podium. Jane came in beaming and wrapped me in a big hug. We were so glad to see each other again.

At last it was time for class. I locked the front door, turned off the lobby lights, put the microphone on, exhaled any nervousness, and stepped into the hot room. The students, all lined up on their mats, turned their heads to watch as I made my way to the podium. As I noticed the expectant look on their faces, I couldn't help but feel like I had walking down the aisle towards Jeffrey on my wedding day.

Standing on the podium, I gazed out at the twenty or so bodies standing in front of me. I said hello and thanked them for coming to my first class, took a breath, and we began.

"Everyone together, toes and heels in one line," I said, my voice bouncing off the walls through the sound system.

In the ninety minutes before me I would do my best to lead this group of students through the class. The Dialogue came tumbling out of my mouth and the bodies responded. Pranayama Breathing felt out of control from the beginning. My rhythm was off somehow, but the students continued anyway. It was as if they were leading me, instead of me leading them. The class seemed to find its rhythm during Half Moon Pose, and I could feel the tension leave my body as I relaxed into saying the words I had spent months memorizing.

When we began Eagle Pose, the third posture in the sequence, I couldn't believe we had already gotten so far. The students before me squatted down, twisting their legs and arms as best they could.

It was so interesting to watch the sea of bodies move from posture to posture and to see the differences, and also the sameness, of everyone at once.

My attention seemed pulled in every direction at once as I concentrated on saying the right words, kept an eye on the room's temperature readings at the humidistat on the podium, and continually checked the clock to make sure I was running on time.

At the first Savasana I was glad to simply stop talking. The silence of the room felt indulgent as I walked to the back of the room and turned the heat up a few degrees as Mara had instructed me. The students would be a little cooler on the floor for the rest of the class, and it was part of the juggling act of teaching to keep the temperature consistent for their practice.

After the final breathing exercise, the students applauded, acknowledging my accomplishment of teaching my first class. As I walked toward the door, I looked back out over the bodies lying in Savasana and felt a surge of relief that everything had gone well, and I knew that this was only the beginning. I couldn't wait to take the podium again. Two days. In two days, I would have another opportunity to teach.

Soon I was teaching an average of five classes a week between my home studio and a second one about forty-five minutes away. It wasn't easy at first to get as many classes as I would have liked. I was a newbie teacher, and other, more experienced teachers had seniority over me when it came to class times. In the beginning, I would teach whenever I could - at six in the morning, at eight at night, it didn't matter. If my phone went off in the middle of the day with a teacher asking for someone to cover a class, I leapt at the chance, hoping to be the first teacher to claim it.

I found the same element of fun and playfulness in teaching that I had when performing. It was never boring. Every time I took the podium to teach was different. Each group of students had their own body of energy. It was fascinating to work within the confines of the class and to try to uplift each individual student as they all worked towards something new within their practices. I quickly learned that a warm smile, a thumbs-up, or a nod and wink could set a first-time student at ease. And I learned that if I was simply myself up on the podium, as vulnerable as that could feel at times, the students could relate to me. There was no need to put on airs or be too demanding, but I always had the expectation that the students would show up and give it their best.

Within a few months I discovered I had developed a reputation for teaching a hard class. When I asked a fellow teacher why the students felt that way, she told me it was because they could tell from the way I watched and paid attention to what was going on in the hot room that I had high expectations for each student.

"I'm only saying the Dialogue," I told her.

"It's the way you say it," she responded. "Not everyone is going to like your class. That's part of teaching. But students generally come around and begin to love the teachers that push them to something new. You're doing great. You want to be known for having a tough class. It's a good thing. It means you care."

It wasn't long after that conversation that I started to offer tips and corrections while teaching class. I was comfortable with the Dialogue at this point and had more to say to help the students go further. It wasn't something I planned for or worked towards, the words simply came out of my mouth while I taught. There is something so satisfying about seeing a posture develop from just a few words spoken in the right way at the right time.

Students began to ask me to take a closer look at their Triangle Pose or Standing Head to Knee and see if I could offer any advice during or after class. Sometimes I would have a line of students with questions. If I didn't know the answer, I would tell them I would look into it and see what answers I could find. I was lucky to have a team of teachers surrounding me that supported my teaching and helped me to grow, patiently answering my questions when I needed advice on how to offer a correction when a student had an injury or was working through pain.

A few months into my teaching, I found that I could no longer practice six days a week. It was too much. Writing projects began to pile up and I never seemed to get ahead or have any kind of time off as I clicked away on my computer between classes. Jeffrey insisted I have at least one day when I was not at the studio, claiming I would be crazy and burned out within the first year if I didn't take a break once a while. Cutting my practice down to four or five days a week seemed to bring a bit of balance to my days, though at first it was hard to admit that I couldn't keep going at my usual pace.

Continuing to practice yoga, and not just teach, was important to me. Each month, when I would tell the studios the times I was available to teach, I made sure that I didn't over schedule myself to the point where I couldn't practice. Students also seemed to relate to the teachers who practiced often. When I rolled out my mat next to them, they could that I too fall out of Standing Bow Pulling Pose and have a hard time with Standing Head to Knee. It helped establish trust between us.

The one thing I was not prepared for my first year of teaching, were the politics of working in a yoga studio. I have come to find that the real drama is not in theater - it's in yoga. From the beginning, I have tried to find an even balance on the ever-shifting ground as my yoga community morphed and reshaped itself.

A few weeks after I returned from teacher training, my home studio announced it was expanding into other types of yoga and would have fewer Bikram classes on the schedule. I was told through an email I could not continue to teach for them if I decided to teach at the new studio that was opening about twenty minutes away, because they thought it was a conflict of interest. This was rough news. I couldn't stay and work at my home studio, perhaps only teaching one or two classes a week, and not work at the new studio, which would allow me to take the podium five or six times a week.

I had some time to think through the situation over the next few months as the studio started to initiate the changes, but I knew in my gut I had to take the leap and leave. In March of 2012, I told them that I would still like to teach for them but that I would be also teaching at the new studio. Since they had decided that wasn't an option, we parted ways and wished each other well. This was not what I had envisioned when I went to teacher training, but I was grateful to have multiple studios to work at (I soon found an additional one) and places to grow as a teacher as well as within my practice.

Other than that, the first year of teaching was an incredible year. Everything was new and exciting. The two studios where I taught were gorgeous and clean with thriving communities and committed studio owners. I loved walking through the doors of each location, absorbing the energy of the good vibes around me as I prepared to teach class.

As I became more and more confident on the podium, I began to tell stories during the Floor Series. It wasn't something I did every day, but if I had a class of students I had already taught a few times that week, I'd find a story that would make them continue to work harder and not tune me out. I'd tell the story a bit at a time in between postures to keep them guessing as to where it might be going. Some of the stories were from my acting career, or about a hike Jeffrey and I had taken that weekend, or just everyday living stories, but I made sure they always related back to yoga and how to live a balanced life. It was fun to share my life with my students in this way. Often the stories would spark conversation after class with students who had a similar story or situation, and through this I was able to get to know each individual in a deeper way. Story time, as one of my students affectionately called it, became a popular part of my class, a treat for those long-time, on-their-mat-every-day students.

My friendship with Jane grew even stronger. We were together all of the time. She made the decision to leave our home studio when I no longer taught there, so that she would be able to take my class or practice right next to me each day. We would work after class on more advanced postures from the Ghosh Lineage or walk our hands down the back wall of the hot room to increase our backward bending, trying to go deeper into postures and work for something new within our practices.

On the home front, the adventure was in finally being home. Seeing Jeffrey every day felt wonderfully decadent. I wasn't thinking about when I would be packing my bags again to head off to the next show. I had a career I was passionate about, and I was able to share my life with Jeffrey and Chandi and to see my family on a regular basis. When I was acting, the focus was on myself. Now as a yoga teacher, the focus was on serving others as best I could - which also, it turns out, served me.

In October of 2013, another studio opened close by, and for a few months I juggled teaching at three studios at once. That winter I decided to take a break from teaching at the studio that was the furthest away, as week after week it would take me over an hour to get there among cars slowed to a crawl on the snow-streaked streets, completely stressing me out as over and over again I barely made it to the studio in time for class. When spring rolled around, I found was that I was booked up between the two closer studios, so I decided to not go back to the third studio, though I missed the owner and that crew of students.

Another shift took place the next year. My community went from one with studios around every corner and tucked into every suburb to one that seemed to be consolidating the most devoted students in just a few areas. One large studio with a huge following closed, so the studios where I was teaching had an influx of new students. Most of them grumbled about the longer drive, but they were grateful to still have a studio where they could keep up their practice.

The next year, my fourth year of teaching, the ground really started to shake. The studio I had given up because of the longer drive announced that it was closing or looking for a buyer. I was shocked. That studio had so many committed students and teachers I couldn't imagine it no longer being around. Not long after that, the studio I had come to call home announced it was being sold too. Studio ownership is hard and exhausting (the work never ends, and it's difficult to make a profit), and I could understand how the passion for running a studio could simply burn out. But, I was crushed. I had taught four or five classes a week and practiced at in that hot room almost every single day.

I thought about buying the studio, and Jeffrey urged me to look into what it would take. He thought that, since I was so passionate about the yoga, studio ownership was an inevitable step for me. But in the end I had to listen once again to what my heart wanted.

Standing behind the desk one morning, awaiting the rush of students to come in for class, I looked around at the high windows with the sun streaming in. I listened to the click of the humidifier kicking in. I took a big inhale and let it go. I knew I wasn't ready to own a studio yet. I had so much more to learn about the yoga and myself before I made a commitment like that.

A few months later it was announced that both studios had been sold to a corporate brand of yoga. The new owners were not yogis. They owned studios as a business investment. They normally did not have Bikram Yoga classes on their schedule, but they planned to keep some of the classes and add in their own brand of yoga as well.

When I told Jeffrey about these new developments on our evening walk with Chandi, I was surprised at his response.

"That is not going to be the right fit for you, Babe. You love Bikram Yoga. These people don't even seem to know what that is," he told me, grabbing my mittened hand in his, and looking my way with a concerned expression, as we both let his words hang in the cold winter air.

He was right. But how could I leave that studio and those students? They had been my every day for the past four years.

I hung on for a couple of months. I did my best to make it work. But the new type of classes added to the schedule had a methodology that contradicted the teachings of Bikram Yoga. I began to feel that the stress and complication of staying outweighed the ties I had to that community. The choice I had to make felt like the one I had made when I first started teaching and had to leave my first studio. I wanted to teach at studios that supported the yoga I loved and taught it with integrity.

I began to teach more classes at the only true Bikram Yoga studio left in my neck of the woods, finding refuge with the teachers and students there that continued to believe in the practice. And a studio on the other side of Chicagoland contacted me to see if I'd be willing to make the trek out their way once a week to teach for them. I committed to drive quite a bit out of my way once again, and fortunately, teaching for that studio turned out to be exactly what I needed that year. The studio shaped me, and continues to shape me, into a better teacher and practitioner, challenging me in ways I need to be challenged.

As I look ahead I am hopeful. My next goal is to get certified to teach an intermediate Ghosh Yoga class, which stems from the same lineage as Bikram Yoga, but makes advanced postures accessible to students that want an extra challenge. I have known for a while that I would head this way, and now I feel that the timing is finally right to move forward with my own education and practice.

I know that I still love Bikram Yoga in its ninety-minute form, and I love to teach it that way, too. I do teach a sixty-minute version of the series a few times a week and have come to enjoy it, though I feel that the students don't get the same benefits that they would receive if they put in that extra half hour. The sixty-minute class is more of a workout than a meditation, but people are busy, and teachers and studios still want to make the yoga accessible, so the sixty-minute version continues to thrive at studios everywhere.

More and more studios are changing their names to something that does not include Bikram Choudhury's name to distance themselves from the controversial figure that he has become. These studios opt to offer Yin Yoga, Hot Vinyasa, and Hot Pilates, as well as Bikram's original hot yoga. With all the changes, I am optimistic that whatever this all morphs into will be a positive thing, and I hope that more and more people find yoga and its healing potential.

I also hope that - though there may not be a lot of Bikram Yoga – only studios that strictly adhere to the ninety-minute class format and the insane love-it-and-hate-it-all-at-once heat - the class still lives on at studios across the globe. For what I do know is this yoga, the original hot yoga, does heal. It embraces every single human body that comes to it in whatever condition that body shows up - no matter if those bodies are sick, or old, or have an injury, or mental illness. It does not matter what addictions those bodies face or trauma they have endured. Everybody who truly commits to this practice will find space - space to breathe and space in the body, mind, and heart - and that space does heal.

Unlocking the studio doors and flipping on the lights, I step into the hot room and feel my shoulders relax as the heat washes over my skin as I check to make sure everything is set for class. Students come in, hands full of mats, towels, and water bottles. I greet each one with a smile. I check in with the sixty-two-year old career woman coming back to the practice after knee surgery. I ask the stressed-out single mom of three how her weekend was and if her little boy is over that cold he had last week. I greet the local policeman who comes to help reduce the stress of his job and to heal an old hip injury that bothers him when he can't make it to the studio. I welcome back the constantly traveling businessman, who just flew in from China and is hitting the studio before he drives home to his family. I greet the Ironman triathlete, the fresh faced teenaged girl with her hair done up in a messy top knot, the friendly couple from India, the Jujitsu fighter that won his match last weekend, and the high school counselor skating in at the last second, coming in straight from school.

It's time for class once again. I walk to the front of the room in silence and climb the three steps to the top of the podium. I look out at the range of students - all standing with their feet together, meeting their own reflections in the mirror - and I am awed at the beauty of so many different skin colors and body types, people from every walk of life that have come together to practice. As I know from my own experience, each student holds inside the promise of a new beginning, of conquering fears, and of being able to do something she or he never thought possible - and I get to watch it all happen as they stand side by side, sweating it out, pushing through the discomfort to find the light in their lives, so they can be the light for others. My heart surges with gratitude for the next ninety minutes. For me, the view from the podium is the best view.

MAT TO MAT CHAT
KAREN

Karen has a one of the best smiles in the world. I would never have known that when I first met her. In fact, I would never have known that within the first three *months* of knowing her, but she does have the best smile. It's one of those smiles that is bright white teeth and affects every part of her face, shining from her big blue eyes that puts you in a better mood when you see it.

When Karen would walk through the doors of the studio at the beginning of her practice I remember thinking, *"Why is this woman so angry?"* Her face was drawn into an exasperated frown, wrinkles lined on her forehead as she handed me her key tag to check her into class, barely mumbling a hello as she headed into the hot room to set up her mat. The same attitude would be carried into class as she worked on each posture, at times wobbling or falling out and then cursing under her breath, avoiding looking in the mirror and when she did it was a huge glare at herself as if to say, "Come on - get it together!" in the most punishing sense of these words.

"I think that was my love/hate relationship I was having with the yoga," Karen admitted to me, grinning from ear to ear with that awesome mega-watt smile. "In the beginning, I was constantly checking the schedule to see who was teaching and if it was someone that would tick me off I would avoid that class. Now I see everybody has their thing. Some teachers hold a posture longer than others, but it all works out in the end - it's ninety-minutes. Sometimes when I'm in class my brain explodes with the thought, '*Hey, that Savasana was **not** twenty-seconds! I haven't gotten one breath in! That was **not** long enough,*' but that's all part of the challenge of the class.

Karen's story is not unlike others in the fact that she stumbled upon her yoga practice by accident, it showing up in her life when she needed it, though her commitment to being fit and healthy started many years before. Finding herself in need of a regular workout routine after having two kids she admits she was huge and unhealthy.

"I remember thinking, '*I'm going to die if I don't do something,*'" she admits.

Starting with a simple walking routine, she found the pounds started dropping off and she was getting healthier. From there she went to the gym.

"I have a pattern of getting into something for a few years and then I would leave it behind for something else," she says.

Eventually, she found herself running and running and running until her knees got so bad the doctor told her she had to quit, explaining to her that being in her late fourties, she was too young for a knee replacement. Karen was preparing for a marathon at the time and was devastated to have to give up that goal.

With the doctor's recommendation she started biking, but it wasn't the same. Headed back to the gym, her now adult daughter wanted to get healthy too and started to join her. They were on the machines, working out when her daughter asked if Karen would ever take the yoga classes the gym offered with her.

"My first thought was, '*Oh no, I don't want to do yoga. My heart rate is **never** going to get up and it will be a waste of time.*' That was my mindset. The balance part of those classes was interesting to me and that was about it. But the goal was to keep my daughter coming to the gym, so we kept doing the yoga classes. Thankfully, we had a great instructor. She was the one that told us about the Bikram Studio and my daughter and I thought we should check it out."

Karen's first class was much like everyone's experience. The teacher on the podium had a slight accent and she found it hard to understand everything at first, so she followed along with the students in front of her, trying to match what their bodies were doing.

Laughing, she recalls, "We were almost through with the Standing Series and I remember looking at the teacher and asking, 'Isn't there an easier way to do this?!!'" Then the student in front of me turned around and went, 'Shhh!' and I thought, 'Oh God, we're not supposed to talk in here.'"

Other than that, it was the heat that got to her the most, as it does most first-time students.

"I remember lying there and thinking, *'It's so hot. How are all of these people staying in the room when it is so hot?'*"

After she completed her first class, she knew she would come back. Karen possesses a fierce motivation to strive to be better than she was the day before, as well as, a never give up personality that is apparent to any teacher on the podium. Nothing stops her from pursuing and conquering her goals which you can tell from the way she approaches each posture.

"Once I figured it out and got used to the heat, I thought, *'I'm not going to give up. I will conquer this if it kills me. I am staying in here. I will die rather than accept defeat.'* And then once you listen to your teachers and realize you simply have to stay in the room, take breaks, listen to your breath... it makes a difference."

When Karen first started practicing, you knew something was going on with her knees. The Floor Series was tough, as many of the postures require you to sit in a kneeling position, and for her, Fixed Firm Pose, or Supta Vijrasana, was the worst of it. She started as most students with knee problems do - sitting up straight in the posture as she allowed her hips to slowly descend to the floor in between her heels, each class getting her a millimeter closer to her goal.

I remember telling her more than a few times she would be able to get into the full expression of that posture some day and to be patient. She would look at me doubtfully, like I had lost my mind, or that the green juice I was always drinking had obviously gone to my brain, and that I had no idea what I was talking about, before she would head out the studio doors.

A year into her practice, on a Saturday morning packed class that had wall to wall yogis crammed into the hot room, Karen went back onto her elbows in the posture and I could see that she would be able to do the full posture that day if I talked her through it.

"Are you ready?" I asked her during the twenty-second Savasana in between sets.

She nodded, we set up the posture, the class went as deep as they could and there Karen was, dropping her head back, tucking her chin into her chest, with her arms over her head grabbing each opposite elbow. And I found myself getting teary eyed at the sight. How amazing to see a student come this far so fast! These moments are not only an unforgettable moment for the student, but for the teacher as well. To experience someone going past what they ever thought was possible for them and proving to themselves that the body can heal and change for the better is pure magic. It is witnessing greatness.

When talking with Karen about this experience she admits, "Even now it's bad. I shouldn't say it's bad, but it's hard. Some days it's easy and some days it's so difficult – but it's like that with all of the postures."

Not long after that Karen, a long-time sky diver, ripped out her rotator cuff. Inspiring to me, to learn that she jumped a minimum of 40 times throughout the summer months in Chicago, I have always been amazed with what this woman takes on in her life.

"It wasn't one thing. It was wear and tear from sometimes hundreds of jumps in a season. One of the tendons completely tore off when I experienced a hard opening of my parachute, where I came down thinking, *'Okay now my shoulder is messed up.'* The other tendons were just worn down from over use. So, the hard opening, which feels like whiplash when it happens, triggered it."

She believes she was able to get back to the studio much sooner than if she had not practiced Bikram Yoga prior to her injury and that she healed quickly because of continuing her practice. It was rough going at first. I could see the frustration on her face and the defeat in her spirit as she tried to regain what she felt was lost when it came to the flexibility and strength of her arm. Though I know that joint will never be the same for her after she had the surgery to repair and clean the tendons involved, she is not the first or the last student that will be able to enjoy a range of motion that the doctors warn their patients may never achieve after rotator cuff injury. In trying to move the body, the body finds a way to safely achieve the motion of the postures when the student has patience and commits to the practice. Within a year after the injury and surgery, Karen was back to normal. Only if you knew what she had been through, would you be able to see it within her practice and her life outside the room.

When talking about her practice she says, "It's still hard today. There are some days I walk in there, and one thing I've learned from all this is I'll be driving in the car thinking, *'I'm feeling great! I'm going to have a great class!'* and then you get in there and you're like get me out of here. And then other days you don't want to go and you have a great class. I have no expectations anymore. There are days where you're like, *'Yes! I'm getting this!'* And then you come in the next day and you realize you didn't have it at all – it's like Day One. But that's what keeps me coming back. It's not the same. When people say they couldn't do the same set of postures every day, I'm like, *'Well the postures are the same, but you don't ever feel the same. There are no two days alike.'* They just don't get it.

Currently, Karen has taken up sailing. She is always trying something new and taking up new interests, learning everything she can about the topic or activity at hand. Admittedly, Karen has a pattern of diving into it, learning everything she can and then moves onto the next activity or event, leaving whatever she had just tackled behind, almost as if she's checked it off a metaphorical list of

Been There, Done That. I recently asked her, "What makes you stick with Bikram Yoga?"

She smiled at me with a knowing expression, blue eyes flashing and said, "I haven't mastered it yet."

We all know none of us ever will. Yoga is never ending and always evolving and there will always be more to learn. It is the study of your Self and we are always changing. I looked at her and said, "Good to know I'll see you in the hot room for the next fifty years," and we laughed.

CHAPTER NINE
BEYOND THE PODIUM

I had been teaching for about a year, and the fall winds had started to blow once again in the Chicago suburbs, when I began to think that there had to be more to teaching yoga. This thought started as something small, but it soon grew into a search for what "more" might even mean. I knew there was more to yoga than the class and the postures, but I had no way to convey that to the students other than to touch lightly on philosophy or mention between postures small ways to live a positive life. Sometimes I would leave the studio wishing I had had more time to explore a correction of a posture with a student. Sometimes I would leave thinking about a story I had told and wishing I had phrased it differently or streamlined it a bit to create greater impact. The ninety-minute time frame of the class seemed restrictive at times as we plowed through each posture towards the final breathing exercise. Also, I wanted to grow and contribute somehow to the overall community of yogis and yoga teachers that surrounded me.

When I went to teacher training in 2011, Bikram Choudhury was already in the news, involved in a copyright lawsuit against a yoga studio for teaching his Beginning Class (twenty-six postures and two breathing exercises) without his authorization. He claimed that the order of the postures was his system and that he should have control over it. I could see both sides to this situation. On the one hand, he was the one to put the class together. But, on the other, these postures had been around for thousands of years. They didn't belong to anyone. So, when I first took the podium as a beginning teacher, I became used to answering questions from students who had seen the story in the news or watched the latest interview with Bikram as he fought and lost his battle. His Dialogue for the class was copyrighted, and that could only be used by teachers who attended his trainings, but the sequence of postures was fair game for anyone that wanted to teach it at their studios.

It was around my one-year anniversary of beginning my life as a teacher that the other stories began to come out. Women were stepping forward to say they had been sexually harassed and even raped by Bikram Choudhury. These allegations tore our community apart. The teacher Facebook groups (where Bikram Yoga teachers usually asked questions of other, more experienced teachers about postures or how to work with students who had various issues or limitations) became forums mainly about one thing: the allegations against Bikram Choudhury. People took sides. Some stood with the women and others stood with Bikram. I stood with the yoga. It had never been about Bikram Choudhury for me. It was about the yoga that I loved to teach and practice. If he had caused harm to other women, then he should face the consequences of his actions.

I scoured the Internet for positive thoughts and places to get inspired about the yoga. There were a few blogs out there, but some didn't post anything regularly and others had been all but abandoned, with no fresh posts for over a year. There was an incredible chat room led by senior teachers that focused on teaching and how to be better at it, but I was looking for something more. I was looking for a voice that would say that this yoga is great and everyone should try it and keep showing up, because it gets better and better.

By January of 2013 I had given up my search. Out for our walk with Chandi one night, bundled up in layers of coats and clothes to insulate us from the numbing chill that is winter in Chicago, I finally told Jeffrey the idea that had been bouncing around in my head for weeks.

"I've been thinking about blogging."

"About yoga?" he asked.

"Mainly about Bikram Yoga. I keep looking for something out there that I can't find," I said. Even as I said it I wondered if I could do it. After all, I had been teaching for only a year. I was a baby teacher. Maybe this idea wasn't meant for me, maybe it was meant for someone else with more experience. "I have no idea if anyone will read it or even care that I'm doing it."

"Why not? You already write. It sounds like an interesting project."

"But I know nothing about blogging. I don't even read blogs," I said. "But I get so frustrated when I read an article online about the twenty-six-and-two, and they warn that it's too dangerous with the high temperature in the room - and it's written by someone that admittedly has never tried the practice. Or a piece that is all about Bikram Choudhury and what's happening for him personally. Where's the article from someone that practices and loves it? Or the story about the person with chronic back pain that is now pain free because they get to the hot room three times a week?"

"Go for it Babe. What have you got to lose?" he asked, patiently letting me talk this out to him and mostly to myself.

"I'm scared that other teachers won't understand why a first-year teacher would do this. Or that they'll think I shouldn't do it."

"Take the chance anyway," he said, grabbing my hand and leaning in to give me a quick kiss.

"I even have a name for the blog," I said, smiling at his encouragement. "For some reason, it came to me a few days ago and it keeps running through my mind on repeat. Views from the Podium. What do you think?"

He liked it. Squeezing my hand twice in confirmation, he smiled at the thought of it.

As we hurried through the cold towards the light of our apartment building ahead, I felt excited at the thought of this new venture. It could be something or it could be nothing, but it was new. It was the "more" I had been looking for.

I began the next morning. I already had a name, but I needed a place for this blog to live. I started looking at my options for blog platforms. I knew people read and even subscribed to blogs, but I wasn't thinking that much about creating some kind of following. I didn't actually read blogs, except for clicking through to an article that someone had posted on Facebook every once in a while, so this all felt brand new.

With ten minutes before I had to leave to go teach class, I quickly scribbled down some thoughts about what my blog would be about. First, of course, it would be about Bikram Yoga. And it would be from the perspective of a new teacher. It would focus on the practice of yoga both in and outside of the hot room. And it had to be positive - no yoga politics or breaking news or gossip. I could tell stories from my life, like I did during class, to teach an idea or thought, but I wanted the blog to sound like it could be coming from any teacher, anywhere.

Later that afternoon, sitting on the couch with my hair still wet from my after-class shower, I started to design the look and feel of the web site. It didn't' take long. In a little under an hour I was set to begin posting - but what would I write about first?

My mind kept going back to a moment in my class that morning. In the middle of Standing Bow Pulling Pose I saw a student in the second row catch her own two eyes in the reflection in front of her. Until this day Claudia had avoided looking forward into the mirror, but instead of looking away, she continued to gaze forward. She didn't have a look of disgust, or disappointment, or even that watch-how-hard-I'm working-over-here look that I so often see from the podium. Instead the gaze back at herself was filled with what looked like compassion and maybe a little bit of wonder at what she was accomplishing in that moment.

Claudia wasn't the first and wouldn't be the last student to do this. It is something I have seen time and again, week after week. In our culture, many of us have been taught not to look too long at ourselves in the mirror in front of other people, so as not to appear vain or over indulgent. I find most students avoid looking at themselves for other reasons though. Most start their practice with a good deal of self-hatred for whatever reason. They may hate their bodies. They may hate their jobs. They may think they will never be good enough for somebody or some experience. It varies. But ultimately, it is a disconnect from the truth of who they are and what they are capable of. I recalled another student, Mary, who had always insisted on practicing in the back row, and then suddenly, just the day before, she had moved her mat to the front of the room to truly get a good look at herself and her practice. Inspired, I smiled and began to write my first post.

I picked apart and edited the post for two days, working on it between other writing projects and trips to the studio to teach or take class. It was fun to write something and not have to assume someone else's voice, as I did when writing projects for my clients. It was something I hadn't done in a long time and it felt luxurious and liberating. When I told Jane what I was doing, she thought the blog was a great idea and said she couldn't wait to read what I had written. This boosted my confidence a bit, knowing that at least one person might actually read it.

While I was teaching class on the second day, I found myself thinking about the post and how I could make it better. This was during the first Savasana, and I looked down at the clock on the podium to realize that maybe I had let the two-minute break go on a little longer than was necessary. As I started the Dialogue back up again, instructing the students into Wind Removing Pose, I told myself to just publish it and let it go. The post would be what it was going to be, and people would either read it or not, and like it or not. I couldn't let it become a distraction. So, that afternoon I hit the publish button, posted the link to my Facebook page, and, with the nervous excitement of having tried something new, walked away from the computer.

The next day at the studio I was surprised to have students stop by the front desk before and after class to tell me they liked the blog post, saying that during class they had thought about what I had written and applied it to their practice. This was what I was hoping for - that I could teach beyond the podium. And it seemed to be working.

From the very beginning my goal in writing the blog has been to inspire students and teachers alike to keep up their practice, because I know how hard that is to do. I hadn't expected to feel as passionate as I do about writing for the blog. Possibly, this passion comes from how the blog has helped me to be honest with myself about my practice and given me time to reflect on my own life.

One of the main benefits of blogging I have found through the years is the connection I have gained with students and teachers around the world. This has helped me to become a better teacher and a better person than I was when I started the blog. I had thought that my students would read the posts, but I had never considered how far-reaching a post could be when it is shared across the Internet by like-minded yogis. It is intimidating at times to see the high-ranking stats of a post, or see that, yes, the United States and Canada seem to like it, but Australia, New Zealand, and Germany are nuts about it. Yogis I might never meet are reading, and that makes me realize how similar we all are. We love this yoga and want to share with others its healing potential.

At first, I published a post every Tuesday morning. I had so many ideas in the beginning, and I kept a running file of thoughts that would jump into my head that I might shape into blog posts. Now, as the years roll by, I publish a post two or three times a month when inspiration strikes. Sometimes, I feel hunted down by a new post, the words connecting in my head and overloading me to distraction until I can find the time to sit down and put them on the page. Other times, it's more of a challenge to get a post done. But, it's always fun. Just as it's always exciting to see new readers find the blog. And I still always feel a bit nervous - and curious - about how each post will do when I send it out into the world, as I did on that first day.

Where are your eyes?

From the Blog: January 23, 2013

The more I teach, the more I see it. A new student comes into the studio ready to face the challenge of their first class, braving the 105-degree heat and forty-percent humidity for the first time. They may be in the back row or, if they're feeling courageous, the second row, beginning their sweaty adventure, following along with the words and watching those in front of them. But the sure-fire way to spot a first-time student in the room is not how they move through the series of postures, just the plain simple fact that they are unable to meet their eyes in the front mirror.

It's kind of interesting in a world of Facebook, Twitter, camera phones, websites and blogs that 9 out of 10 people that take their first Bikram Yoga class can barely look at themselves in the eyes. You would think that we would have gotten used to looking at ourselves at this point. But to look at ourselves with no make-up, hair pulled back, red-faced, sweaty, and quite vulnerable while surrounded by others is a challenge that even the most experienced Bikram yogi struggles with at times.

To accept where we are today - what we look like, how we feel - is an incredible lesson to learn through our

163

practice. Acceptance does not mean apathy or feeling hopeless. It means knowing that, once you entered the doors of the studio, you have altered the path of your health, well-being, and therefore, your life. By taking that first class (no matter how grueling it may feel at the time) you have to accept where you are today, but you already know that there is more to your tomorrows.

One of my favorite things about being a Bikram Yoga instructor is seeing that first-time student avoid their eyes in the mirror and then little by little, class after class, come to fall in love with their own reflection. To have a student that always chooses the back row finally drag their mat to the front of the room, unapologetic for what their practice may be at that time and taking ownership of their health, self-esteem and overall wellness, is a powerful moment in the course of their yoga practice

So, next time you hit the hot room, ask yourself, "Where are your eyes?" You may realize that they are everywhere but in the mirror. No worries — just noticing a habit in your practice is the first step to changing it. And remember — those mirrors aren't meant for you to spend ninety minutes telling yourself everything that's wrong with you or what you would like to change. Make it an opportunity to truly focus on all of the many things that make up the wonderful, thrilling, positive aspects of your own personal journey.

MAT TO MAT CHAT
CHRISTI

Christi was better than most at the beginning of her practice. She seemed to have an eye and ear for the details and mastered the grips and shapes of the postures within a handful of classes. Most of the time her face was relaxed, and her practice had a quiet concentration about it. The only time she became flustered or overwrought was when we came to Triangle Pose. I could tell she hated that posture the first time I saw her in class. Her face lost its composure, her brow furrowed, and her jaw tightened in determination. When we hit the second set, she took a seat, looking at the floor in defeat and waiting for the posture to pass.

Tall and curvy, Christi had always been up and down with her weight. At times she was able to get herself down to 118 pounds, and even when she wasn't restricting her diet, she would have a panic attack if the scale weighed her in over 126 pounds. As with all too many of us, the number on the scale defined who she thought she was. After having three kids she relaxed a bit (her weight about

190), but once she knew she wouldn't have any more children she went right back to working out regularly, restricting her food, and beating herself up mentally every day for carrying the extra weight.

When Christi first started yoga, she was coming off of three long years committed to running, an activity she never enjoyed but that she continued to pursue anyway.

"Running was killing me! I had a lot of friends who ran, and they were always pushing me to give it a shot. I liked the sense that I could plan. I liked the training of it very much. I thought that if I did it long enough it would grow on me, but it never did. And then I thought about the amount of time I was giving it - out on a run for two or three hours. I was not enjoying it, and my knees were starting to bother me."

Once she had started her yoga journey, Christi was committed. "I decided to take three weeks to see if I really liked it. I went a lot. I wanted to complete thirty classes in the first thirty days - I did twenty-six or twenty-seven. I remember the instructors saying to me, 'You must really like this yoga!' And I remember thinking, 'I'm not sure that I do.'"

Before she began she had studied the Bikram Yoga poses online and thought, "I can do this. I can do that." But the actual experience wasn't so easy. "It's different doing it all sweaty and melting and holding the postures as long as you have to hold them. The first time I took the class I was just trying to breathe. I was sweating and extremely uncomfortable, but I did come back, so there must have been something about it."

But she kept on. She became a regular fixture at the studio, tucked into the back corner, second row of the hot room, one of the 5:30 a.m. crew. Triangle Pose continued to challenge her. Some days she would be able to hold the pose, exiting out of the posture with a huge megawatt smile, relishing her accomplishment. On others, her feet would start to slide apart, her rib cage start to collapse; she would take a seat, but she would rise again, once she had recovered, to tackle the challenge of the posture again and again.

About a year into her practice Christi found herself feeling a bit adrift and unfocused. She decided to give herself a personal thirty-day challenge, thinking it was a good way to celebrate her year in the hot room and knowing that a challenge always motivated her. After she had begun the studio announced that it would be holding a studio-wide thirty-day challenge, so she decided to keep going, doubling her challenge to sixty days. Then she thought, why not make it an even hundred? One hundred classes in one hundred days, a nice, tidy number and a defined endpoint. She liked the sound of it.

As she worked toward her goal, I checked in with her periodically to see how she was feeling. Was she sore? Did she need any tips to get her through? Strong and confident, she kept on, day after day.

Then one day I found her sitting in the women's changing room. The 9:30 a.m. class was still in progress in the hot room across the lobby. I sat down next to her.

"I feel awful," she confessed.

I asked where she was in her challenge.

"About half way there."

"So, you left the room. Congratulations!" I smiled.

She glared at me. Usually, I am a teacher who encourages students never to leave the hot room during class, and here I was making light of it.

"Don't be so hard on yourself. It's humbling to leave the room. It can feel devastating to someone as devoted as you are to the practice, but it's also not the end of the world. You don't need to be perfect to practice this yoga - you need to be you. And you needed to leave today and take care of yourself. You did what you had to do for you without caring what the teacher or the rest of the students thought. That's your yoga for the day. Tomorrow is another day. You'll make it through. You showed up, you did your practice, let this one go."

She looked at me with disbelief. And relief. "Have you ever left the room?"

"In teacher training I had to leave a few times, and what I learned from that was compassion for my own journey. It's not a bad lesson to learn. It's okay not to be perfect. In fact, it's impossible to be perfect at yoga."

Just a few days from the end of her challenge, Christi came out of class, glowing and dripping, sat down on the bench in front of me, and announced that she had had a huge breakthrough the day before.

"What posture?" I asked.

"All of them."

After Christi completed her hundred-day challenge I asked her to put into words the experience she had on that day. She wrote:

"When I looked in the mirror, under those glaring, unforgiving fluorescent lights, I looked into my own eyes and I saw acceptance. Then I saw forgiveness. And then I started to cry. In that moment, I realized that I'd never actually looked at myself. I would avoid eye contact with my reflection at all costs. I always have. I'd just let my eyes kind of glaze over and lose focus as if I were seeing myself from beneath a veil. And just like that, the veil was gone. I am convinced that was the first time I saw *me*.

"I learned that my body is more than just the sum of its parts. It is a machine - a twenty-four-hour-a-day, miracle-producing machine. I began to be more conscientious of the fuel I was providing it, because I had to. Better food choices, better hydration, better sleeping habits. After a while, I stopped seeing myself as a mass of perceived flaws and only saw the 'machine.' I began to acknowledge how fortunate I was that this piece of equipment was mine and that it deserved my respect. In losing my preoccupation with my reflection, I began to see the real me."

This realization has helped Christi discuss body image with her children and serve as an example to them on how to respect and treat their own bodies. Each of her daughters has rolled out a mat next to Christi, not sure yet if they like the yoga, but knowing that it plays an important role in their mom's life.

And her Triangle pose after a year and a half of devoted work in the hot room? It is as solid as the rest of her practice. Although she still dislikes the posture, her face no longer shows it, and she has a calm, cool demeanor that says, "I've got this."

When discussing the posture with me, Christi admitted, "Lately the Universe is telling me I'm ready for Triangle. I was online the other day and saw a video of Bikram (Choudhury) doing Triangle, and he said, 'Hips forward.' It was the gesture of the hips in that video that clicked with me. You've told me that a billion times, but I wasn't ready to hear it. Then two days later I saw a video of Joseph Encinia teaching Triangle. I hear, "Don't collapse, or lift up, stretch up" every day in class and always thought it wasn't directed at me. His demo made me I realize I collapse through the ribcage. I'm Queen Collapse! The next day, I was at the 4:15 p.m. class, and I forgot how much more flexible I am later in the day. I felt fantastic. I put the hips forward and went for it. I can't believe how much bringing the hips forward made a difference."

She sometimes wishes she could have started her yoga practice twenty years ago or made some of the connections sooner. "But I'm also glad that it took a while, because you do appreciate it when you finally arrive at your goal and get closer to achieving the posture. I believe a pose is more than just a pose - it runs parallel to your life, the way you think, and the relationships you keep. I didn't believe that before, but I do believe that now."

In Defense of Bikram Yoga

From the Blog: May 17, 2016

Some people will love this post and some people will absolutely hate it. Some people will only read the first couple of paragraphs and then click on to the next thing, claiming I am awesome, or that I suck, or that I have no idea what I'm talking about. That's okay. I write this blog for you, but I also write this blog for me.

Lately I've been thinking that maybe I am simply stuck in my old ways. I fell in love with Bikram Yoga over ten years ago and am still one of the practice's biggest fans. I have tried other types of yoga. I *do* practice other types of yoga when I get the chance, but Bikram Yoga is still one of my favorite things in life.

Over the past couple of years, I've watched as the community of Bikram Yogis has shifted and evolved. There was no way that it couldn't. Change is inevitable and is not a bad thing. I think it's interesting to see studios embracing other types of yoga and hot Pilates classes. I am intrigued by, and can't wait to take, the new intermediate classes that are popping up at studios here and there. I believe all yoga is good yoga and that anyone that starts up a regular yoga asana practice is a brave, brave soul on the journey of a lifetime.

That being said, I hope that beyond my lifetime there is still Bikram Yoga available and accessible to those who need it. I hope that there is still a hot room where future yogis can all get crazy sweaty and red faced, lined with mirrors so that they can grin at themselves as they collectively create that pitter patter as the sweat drips from, well... *everywhere* under fluorescent lights.

"Why should I care?" you might ask. We'll be long gone. Who cares what happens when we are no longer here anymore? And I tell you this. I was a mess before Bikram Yoga (Hot Traditional Hatha Yoga, the twenty-six and two, or whatever the heck you all are calling it these days) came into my life. I was also a mess for quite a few years after I established a regular practice. I had low self-esteem, body-image issues, and few positive relationships. I had back issues, hip issues, chronic skin issues, allergy issues, and sciatic pain at twenty-eight years old. I struggled to fit in anywhere and connect with anyone. I had a brick wall built around me that needed to be chiseled away before I could truly live. And though I do not say that Bikram Yoga was the only thing that cured me of all of this stuff, it definitely had a major impact.

Taking the podium each day to teach class, I am inspired how this yoga brings together people from every walk of life. I look out at my students and see every possible skin color and body shape imaginable. There are students that barely scrape by financially week after week practicing next to the extremely affluent. Dog lovers practice next to cat lovers. Addicts next to trendy moms. Someone dealing with the task of trying to lose a hundred pounds next to an Ironman Triathlete. And all of them feel as if they have accomplished a great deal when they step out of the hot room — because they have.

You might think that this is no big deal. Every yoga class does this, doesn't it? Well, no. In most traditional yoga studios, you will find that there are different levels of classes. If you are just starting out, you may take Level 1 Hatha Yoga. If you are broken in some way, you take Restorative. If you are a rock star yogi, you can take a two-hour Level 3 Power Vinyasa. There is a separation and grouping that happens, in which different folks show up at different times and head to separate rooms to which they belong at the moment.

In Bikram Yoga, everyone belongs. Every posture can be modified to start individual students out where they are at that time in their lives, to set them on the path and get them ready to be transformed in one way or another. We all get to do it together. The person trying to grab his foot for Standing Bow Pulling Pose is getting the same benefits as the person next to him rocking the standing splits in the same posture. Though I love a good Sun Salutation, I also know how impossible it would be for some of my students to accomplish a good Downward Dog or Chaturanga without possibly hurting themselves.

I embrace all yoga, but Bikram Yoga has my heart. Sometimes when there is so much venom around a subject out there in the media we need to shine a light. Bikram Yoga is a healing therapy for millions of souls out there in the world, and I am grateful for the studios that keep it going and honor the sequence, the heat, and the techniques of this type of yoga. And if you haven't tried it, I urge you to take at least one class. Especially, if you are out there saying we are all crazy and that it's too hot, and you should never lock your knee. Be open to every method and recognize we all have different paths. If it's not for you, cool. It's tough stuff no matter where you are physically or mentally, but recognize it has value for those that it was meant for. I would not be who I am today without this practice, and I certainly wouldn't want to be who I was before it. It gave me confidence, love for my body and myself, and a community of people that are a constant inspiration. For me, it made life great.

ACKNOWLEDGMENTS

This book would never have come to be without the constant prodding, pushing, and overall, love and support from my husband, Jeffrey. He was the one that said, "It's not a blog, it's a book. Get started." Jane Hill has been my rock for long before I started writing this book, but was the friend I needed when I had those writer moments of believing that what I created was a disaster that no one would read. She has read countless versions of my first chapter and believed in every one of them, giving me the confidence to keep plugging along and getting it finished. Finding Sam Sherman, my editor, was a defining moment over the past three years of trying to get all the pieces to fit into place. She shone a light on everything that was working and not working and guided me to shape this book into something that was greater than what I had originally envisioned. To the students that shared their time and their real-life yoga story with me - David, Christi, Claudia, Amy, and Karen - I am grateful for your candor and your trust that I would translate your interview into the story you wanted to convey. To my Mom, the original editor of the blog, who always sends me supportive texts and listened to me talk on and on about the process of putting this book together, I could never express how much gratitude and love I have for you. To my Dad, who always made me feel like I could do anything with my life. Thank you for always supporting my every dream and giving me the courage to move forward and make them happen. I love you. To Bikram Choudhury, Rajashree Choudhury, and every teacher that has helped to bring this yoga to the lives of others to affect positive change – thank you. To the studios that have supported and shared the blog with their students, thank you for letting me, even in the smallest way, be a part of your community. And to the students that asked me how the book is going every time they saw me, week after week, for three years – your interest, passion, and enthusiasm for the yoga, the blog, and the possibility of this book, made it actually happen. You were, and are, the driving force behind my work as a teacher, student, and as a writer. Thank you for giving me a space in your life and being my light on a daily basis.